RUN YOUR FAT OFF

Running Smarter for a Leaner and Fitter You

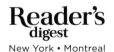

Jason R. Karp, PhD

Reader's
digest

New York • Montreal

Photo Credits: Cover by shapecharge/Getty Images; page 20 (left) by Luke Freedom Hansen; page 20 (right) courtesy of Joshua Snow Hansen; page 46 (right) courtesy of Jessica Skarzynski; page 46 (left) by Michael Reccoppa; pages 51–56 courtesy of the author; page 79 by Jonathan Evans; page 114 courtesy of Roger Lyszczynski; page 143 by Michelle Haub; page 175 courtesy of Jen Hudson Mosher; page 200 by Matthew Shupp; page 215 courtesy of Mark Falkingham; page 228 by Jamie Dickerson of J.Dixx Photography.

LIBRARY of CONGRESS CATALOGING in PUBLICATION DATA
Names: Karp, Jason, author.
Title: Run your fat off : running smarter for a leaner and fitter you /
Jason R. Karp, PhD.
Description: New York, NY : Reader's Digest, [2017] | Includes index.
Identifiers: LCCN 2016040798 (print) | LCCN 2016048681 (ebook) |
ISBN 9781621453352 (paperback) | ISBN 9781621453369
Subjects: LCSH: Running—Training. | Runners (Sports)—Nutrition. |
Reducing exercises. | BISAC: HEALTH & FITNESS / Weight Loss. |
SPORTS & RECREATION / Running & Jogging. | HEALTH & FITNESS / Exercise.
Classification: LCC GV1061 .K386 2017 (print) | LCC GV1061 (ebook) |
DDC 796.42071—dc23
LC record available at https://lccn.loc.gov/2016040798

ISBN 978-1-62145-335-2

We are committed to both the quality of our products
and the service we provide to our customers.
We value your comments, so please feel free to contact us.

Reader's Digest Trade Publishing
44 South Broadway
White Plains, NY 10601

For more Reader's Digest products and information, visit our website:
www.rd.com

Printed in China

1 3 5 7 9 10 8 6 4 2

ALSO BY JASON R. KARP, PHD

The Inner Runner

14-Minute Metabolic Workouts

Running a Marathon For Dummies

Running for Women

101 Winning Racing Strategies for Runners

*101 Developmental Concepts & Workouts
for Cross Country Runners*

How to Survive Your PhD

CONTENTS

◆ ◆ ◆ ◆ ◆

ACKNOWLEDGMENTS

This book would not have been written if not for many people, primary among them my agent, Grace Freedson. Through nearly 9 years of working together, you have responded to every phone call and every email. I am very thankful for your understanding of my persistent personality and for your belief in me. Without you, my work would likely be relegated to a blog read by only a few people.

There are a number of other people I'd also like to thank:

My twin brother, Jack Karp—my greatest writing inspiration—for your insightful comments on the first draft and for not making too much fun of me for writing a weight-loss book. You are the most talented writer I know. You inspire me every day to be a better writer and to tirelessly work at the craft until I get it right.

Andrea Au Levitt, senior editor at *Reader's Digest,* for your thorough feedback that helped shape this book into something that can help millions.

The rest of the team at *Reader's Digest,* including deputy editor Jim Menick, sales and marketing director Kim Gray, and especially cover designer Marti Golon.

Jonathan Little, for planting the seed in my mind of writing a weight-loss book a long time ago. Your no-nonsense, "just get out the door and run" attitude and perspective on life is always welcomed and always sheds light on what's important.

Dominique Adair, one of the smartest and well-read nutritionists I know, for your nutritional expertise and contributions, including the delicious meals and recipes that appear in the *Run Your Fat Off* meal plan. A self-proclaimed nerdy nutritionist, you may be the only person who can convince me to stop eating Froot Loops.

The amazing people who shared their inspiring weight-loss stories that enrich this book: Janel Evans, Mark Falkingham, Joshua Snow Hansen, Mark Haub, Roger Leszczynski, Jen Hudson Mosher, Sarah McDowell Shupp, and Jessica Skarzynski. I hope your stories inspire others to get off the couch and run to become both a better and lighter version of themselves.

The many scientists whom I have studied under and with, for teaching me how to think like a scientist and interpret research with a critical eye. It is because of your influence that I am able to navigate the muddy waters of the weight-loss industry, circumvent the diet propaganda, and search for the truth rather than be swayed by hyperbole and fads.

All my friends, both in person and in social media, for understanding the sacrifices that must be made to write books.

WARM-UP

A **NUMBER OF YEARS AGO,** I was working as a personal trainer in a gym and talking to one of the members as she rode a stationary bike alongside her workout buddies. As I explained how she and her friends could get more out of their workouts, I sensed that she wasn't listening. Maybe she didn't care for the advice of a young, scrawny-looking runner in cotton sweats. Maybe she was just focused on her workout. A few days later, I saw her again as I was about to go for a run. Seeing me for the first time in my running shorts, she enthusiastically asked, "How can I get legs like yours?" Smiling, I joked, "So, you want me for my body rather than for my mind?" Everyone wants nice legs.

For many people, running seems unnecessary or even silly. You put one foot in front of the other and run until you don't feel like running anymore, and you finish in the same place where you started. In our sit-down society, people don't do that. We drive everywhere with GPS devices built into our cars. We sit in front of a screen all day at a desk job and then spend the rest of the day staring at a smaller screen in the palm of our hands. But just because we don't need to run doesn't mean we shouldn't. Runners instinctively know this. Runners know that there is more to life than technology and Twitter feeds. They understand, perhaps better than anyone, that physical effort is the path to a slimmer, healthier, and more fulfilling life. I have always believed that if everyone ran (or at least walked) 5 miles per day, we would eradicate obesity and drastically reduce heart disease. The world would be a better (and slimmer) place if everyone ran.

Running connects you to your body and is perhaps the best expression of your physicality. That's why I deeply believe that running is for *everyone*. Through running, you fulfill your destiny as a physical being, and on the foundation of a fitter physical being, you can build a better life.

Running must become who you are rather than something you do. But that won't be a problem, because once you start running, it becomes addictive. Most runners would agree that no other activity can take the place of running. Even nonrunners have heard of the runner's high. If an ideal form of exercise exists, runners already know what it is and they are already doing it. I think perhaps the reason lies in the simplicity of running—it is just you and the freedom of your movement. To run faster or longer, there is nothing to overcome but yourself. Running is a chance to try.

> " THROUGH RUNNING, YOU FULFILL YOUR DESTINY AS A PHYSICAL BEING, AND ON THE FOUNDATION OF A FITTER PHYSICAL BEING, YOU CAN BUILD A BETTER LIFE."

To make an effort. There's an opportunity for every individual, from the beginner to the Olympian, to try.

Running connects you to your effort. There is a direct relationship between how hard you try and how fast your feet move across the ground. You can choose to challenge yourself on any given day, at any given moment during your runs. You can make your slow runs slower, your fast runs faster, your long runs longer. Running enables you to push yourself past limits you thought you had. As a human, you have the unique capacity—central to who you are as a human—to imagine yourself different than you are, better than you are. You can *imagine* a future for yourself that does not yet exist. You can *imagine* who you want to be. You can *imagine* yourself thinner. You can *imagine* yourself a runner.

When you run to lose weight, you learn about yourself. You learn the effort it takes. You learn what it means to do more, to be more. The journey forces you to shut up, stop complaining, and stop making excuses for why you can't do it. Running teaches you how to give more of yourself. And you come out the other end of the work a stronger, more confident, more capable person, knowing that when the going gets tough, the tough inside of you really *can* get going. When you believe you can accomplish anything, you are no longer timid or scared of pursuing something, because your running has empowered you to be bolder.

Humans evolved to run, especially long distances. Long before the beginning of modern civilization, our ancestors, starting with the apelike *Australopithecus*, raced through woodlands and prairies, chasing wild animals to feed their families. Although humans fare rather poorly compared to other animals when it comes to all-out sprinting (the fastest speed achieved by a human is 23.3 miles per hour, compared to the nearly 70 miles per hour achieved by a cheetah), we are among the best long-distance runners. Our ability to run long distances—and run down faster but less-enduring animals to death—enabled our early ancestors to provide food for their families and thrive as a species. Darwin's survival of the fittest in its most literal form.

Millions of years later, running has become a part of our culture. We witness the joy on a baby's face when he or she takes his or her first tentative steps and we document the occasion. A few years later, schoolchildren discover the freedom that running confers as they race each other on playgrounds across the country, showing off their speed to each other during recess. When those children grow up, they become part of a society in which millions of people run for fitness and train for races. There are thousands of running clubs, clinics, and races all over the United States and the world. Twenty million people run a race in the United States each year. Humans' ability to endure is so rooted in our DNA that when people start running, they inevitably gravitate to run longer and longer distances. Indeed, the marathon is viewed by many runners as the holy grail and has become a popular item on many people's bucket lists. Something special happens when we run and walk on two legs. Bipedal movement is a form of locomotion that makes humans unique from nearly all other animals.

I started running on two legs 44 years ago, soon after I started walking, although it wasn't until fifth grade, during the Presidential Physical Fitness Tests I did in elementary school, that I discovered that I had some talent. Two of the tests were the 50-yard dash and 600-yard run. I ran the 50 in 7.3 seconds and the 600 in 2 minutes, 1 second. I wasn't the quickest in my class. But I was close. I became a runner, and there was no turning back. Some things, once they get started, are impossible to stop.

Nonrunners tend to think that running is hard or boring, and at first it often is. When they start to run, their knees hurt, they get a side ache, they breathe so heavily they feel like their lungs are going to explode. They think, "I'm not a runner. Running is for *those* people." You know who *those* people are—the ones with bionic knees, who have no body fat, who can seemingly eat whatever and however much they want, and who gather for pasta parties and talk about foreign-sounding things like PRs and fartleks and mile splits. But, damn, they're thin with sculpted legs and a spring to their step! Don't you wish you looked and felt like that? That woman in the gym admiring my legs sure did.

Guess what? You *can* look and feel like that. There are many ways to lose inches from your waistline, get a sculpted butt, and even lower your cholesterol and blood pressure. You don't *need* to run for that. But running is one of the most effective means for doing so. On a minute-by-minute basis, running burns more calories than any other exercise, with just one exception: cross-country skiing. But cross-country skiing, as great as it is, requires a high level of skill and can only be done in the snow. Running, which is second only to walking as the most popular exercise in the world, is an inherent skill that can be refined with some practice and is accessible to everyone in the world at any time of the year. Running is the most logical physical activity for weight loss. Even a half hour of running burns more calories than a full hour of most other types of exercise, including swimming, cycling, and weight lifting. And because the weight-bearing nature of running is dangerous for an overweight body, your body acts to get rid of weight fast to protect your joints from damage. So if you want to lose weight and keep it off for the rest of your life, it pays to become a runner. Or at least someone who runs.

"IF YOU WANT TO LOSE WEIGHT AND KEEP IT OFF FOR THE REST OF YOUR LIFE, IT PAYS TO BECOME A RUNNER. OR AT LEAST SOMEONE WHO RUNS."

When it comes to weight loss, people continue to search for what's new. Running, while as old as the human race itself, is new because it has been largely neglected by fitness trainers, weight-loss experts, and publishers. Few other books or programs are centered on running for weight loss. How ironic and awesome it is that an activity so historic, so integral to our evolution and embedded in our civilization, can be looked at in a new way, for a new purpose. Our ancient ancestors ran to get food; now, we run to get away from what food does to our waistlines. And we run to find ourselves.

There is something unique about runners' approach to running and life—and their search for meaning in their running and life—that distinguishes them from all other people who exercise. My own running life has led me to this moment, led me to share how running is the unexplored path to weight loss, vitality, and health. Running, regardless of how slowly or fast it is done, has the power to change people's lives. When you run, you are raw and vulnerable, with nothing to protect you except your own will and courage. Physical effort taps into something visceral in you. It's animalistic. It's powerful. You feel it in a way you don't feel other things. It's easy to get caught up in the moment. When you run, it can bring you to places you never thought possible. And that's why you'll get results with *Run Your Fat Off*.

I have a friend who used to tell me that if I wrote a weight-loss book, it should be one page long. After all, weight loss ultimately comes down to burning more calories than you consume. So that's all I really need to tell people. Run a lot, eat less, and you'll lose weight. While there is much truth to that, it's obviously not that simple, otherwise everyone would be thin.

To be honest, I get annoyed at all the different types of weight-loss programs and diets. The creators of these diets would have the public believe that weight loss is a complicated problem that only their program can solve. Everyone acts like they have come up with a brilliant diet that no one has ever thought of. Losing weight shouldn't be this complicated. Where did all of these diets come from?

In his 2004 TED Talk, Malcolm Gladwell told the story of Dr. Howard Moskowitz, the market researcher who revolutionized the food industry by proposing that the people at the Pepsi company shouldn't spend their time researching and trying to develop the perfect Pepsi; they should develop the perfect Pepsi*s*. As Gladwell explained, Moskowitz brought this idea to other food companies, including Prego, the makers of spaghetti sauce. Moskowitz convinced Prego, as he had done with Pepsi, that having multiple flavors and textures of spaghetti sauce would sell more spaghetti sauce than having just one or two "perfect" options. People like variety more than they like perfection. People have varied tastes and moods and personalities that influence their choices. Perhaps you prefer smooth marinara spaghetti sauce because you are a calm, traditional person. Perhaps you prefer spicy arrabbiata spaghetti sauce because you like to live on the wild side. The specific type of spaghetti sauce you choose when you are standing in the spaghetti sauce aisle in the supermarket doesn't really matter; what matters is that you have a *choice* of which spaghetti sauce to buy. There are dozens of different diets for precisely the same reason.

Diets used to be obsessed with universals, searching for a single set of rules that govern the way all of us eat and behave. But that didn't work because losing weight is not a straightforward problem to solve. Most people who lose weight by going on a diet regain most, if not all, of the weight. Yet people keep coming up with new diets, hoping they will become fads and sell stuff. That none of these diets can agree on the most effective way to lose weight is proof enough that there is no universal magic diet bullet, just as there is no universal truth in spaghetti sauce.

The reason why diets fail and have been ineffective at ameliorating America's obesity epidemic is because they are not sustainable. You can't tell people to stay away from sugar and expect that to be a sustainable strategy. Diets are not designed to be sustainable. They are designed to make money.

The books that advertise their "revolutionary" plans on their covers during which you'll "lose up to 10 pounds in 10 days" don't tell you what happens after those 10 days. Most diets are short-term fixes to a long-term problem. If you start a diet thinking it's going to be short-term, you've already failed. I'll be the first to admit that the *Run Your Fat Off* plan is not revolutionary. I didn't invent running, although I wish I had. The *Run Your Fat Off* plan is different because running is not a short-term weight-loss strategy; it is a lifestyle that is *very* sustainable. Whether you are a beginner, intermediate, or advanced runner, the *Run Your Fat Off* plan will work if you stick with it.

> **" IT IS, PERHAPS, WHAT ISAAC NEWTON HAD IN MIND WHEN HE DEVELOPED HIS FIRST LAW—A BODY IN MOTION STAYS IN MOTION."**

One of the many reasons why running is so effective for sustained weight loss is that it gives you a chance to pursue a tangible goal apart from the weight loss itself—to finish a race. That's why it's so common for people who run to lose weight to enter a race. No other weight-loss method offers that extrinsic reward. There are no diet leagues or exercise DVD competitions you can enter. With running, there's a 5K, 10K, half marathon, or marathon (or races of other distances) on practically every weekend in the United States. When you choose a race to train for, the weight loss becomes a byproduct of the training you do to prepare for the race rather than the center of your focus.

Running, because of its lifestyle and its community, is a

long-term solution to weight loss. It is, perhaps, what Isaac Newton had in mind when he developed his first law—a body in motion stays in motion. People don't become runners for only 6 or 12 weeks; they become runners for a lifetime because they get caught up in the lifestyle and the community. Losing weight may be what gets you started running, but it won't be what keeps you doing it. When you run, you become part of a group that is larger than yourself. You become part of a brotherhood or a sisterhood. You become part of a movement. You become part of an experience. Runners—and running—are everywhere.

So I wrote a book about running and weight loss, and added 235 pages to my friend's one-page suggestion. I admit, writing this book has made me a little anxious, because I never saw myself writing a weight-loss book. I wondered if readers would be able to relate to me because I've never been overweight myself. I've been a competitive runner nearly all of my life. I've always eaten anything I want, believing that running will take care of my waistline. And it has. I have been running 6 days per week, every week, since I was in sixth grade. I don't follow a specific meal plan. And I always eat dessert, especially if it contains chocolate.

But I have coached many runners over the years, from complete beginners to Olympic Trials qualifiers. Many of those beginners didn't think they could run. Many were intimidated by running, and many were overweight. I have spent years researching the effects of running on carbohydrate and fat metabolism, the cardiovascular physiology of runners, nutritional strategies for optimal running performance, and the best ways to train the physiological factors of running, among other things. And I have developed the most effective running workouts for losing weight. Based on my combination of practical training experience and academic research, I can promise you that if you follow this plan, you will get the results you want. Whether you have never run in your life, are morbidly obese, like going to the gym but hate the treadmill, run occasionally, have a few or many pounds to lose, or are a regular runner who wants to lose weight to run faster, this book is for you.

You really *can* run. And if you already run, you really can run more and run smarter and better than you do now. Is it going to be difficult? Probably. Is it going to be worth it? You bet it is.

To lose weight, you're going to have to make a big change in your life. You're going to have to be willing to do the work. And you're going to have to stop eating so much because that's what got you fat in the first place. Too many people quit running before they get to the point where the effort becomes effortless. And for those who already run, it's too easy to grab another slice of pizza or a few more French fries because they think they can get away with it. Running is hard and losing weight is hard. But, guess what? Life is hard. Just because running is hard doesn't mean you should shy away from it. The trick is learning how to deal with the hard parts so you can enjoy the fun parts and see the results you want. It is precisely in working through the difficulty that you reap the benefits that count the most.

When you reject all of the popular media nonsense about fad diets, accept that losing weight is hard work, and then you get to work—*that* is true personal freedom, and that is what is going to make you feel wonderful. You'll look in the mirror and see the results of the new you. Committing to running creates a habit not only of running but of all the traits that it takes to be successful in all areas of your life, including discipline, devotion, perseverance, and attitude. You'll need all of those traits to lose weight and keep it lost. It takes a lot of discipline and devotion to head out the door to run despite the weather, your mood, your kids, or your busy schedule. And then do it again tomorrow. And tomorrow. And tomorrow. When you develop these traits, you open the door to new possibilities. Despite our instant gratification society, humans evolved to persevere. It's why running a marathon has become so popular around the world. Humans like the results that come from perseverance. So don't quit just because you haven't lost 5 pounds this week. Patience is more than just a virtue when it comes to weight loss; it is your pathway to success.

The plan I lay out in this book represents an opportunity for you to make a change in your life for the better. This plan is not a fad. It is a way of life that is based on science and on what it really takes to lose weight and keep it off for the rest of your life. This book doesn't sugarcoat things, doesn't have pictures of pretty people doing abdominal exercises with six-pack abs, doesn't give you false promises like "lose 10 pounds in 2 weeks" like so many others in the fitness and weight-loss industry do. If you commit to this plan, you will not only see results, you will also be proud of committing to a goal and not being satisfied with mediocrity. It's up to you to make the change.

This book took more pages than I would have liked, but it works. By the way, if you want to know the one page I would have written if I followed my friend's one-page book idea, turn to page 39.

CHAPTER 1

Running for Weight Loss

**"I DIDN'T HAVE A VISION OF THE FUTURE
AND IT DIDN'T HELP THAT I BUSTED THE CROTCH
OUT OF MY GRADUATION GOWN."**

ON THE WEBSITE of the Bugout Run, there is a quote by Lailah Gifty Akita: "Every action in the present prepares us for the future." It is central to the philosophy of the Bugout Run, a series of endurance challenges that combine the worlds of running, wilderness survival, and emergency preparedness. Thirty-four-year-old Joshua Snow Hansen is one of the founders of and participants in the events, which showcase running as liberating, fostering self-reliance, and bringing out our survival instinct.

That Joshua founded, much less takes part in, the Bugout Run is rather shocking. He once weighed 402 pounds. At that weight, it's safe to say he wasn't prepared for any emergencies except for a trip to the emergency room. As a child growing up in Bountiful, Utah, he never wanted to leave the familiar comfort of home. Even getting him to go to school was a challenge. "I couldn't understand why my mother would separate me from home and from her,"

Joshua says. "Why would she rip me away from a place where I felt safe, loved, and able to be myself and put me into situations and places where I felt vulnerable, unsure, and alone?" There were often tears as his mother dropped him off at school. "It wasn't easy on either of us," he says.

Interestingly, Joshua was raised in a large family that valued self-reliance, preparedness, and creativity. Throughout his life, he has been fascinated with natural disasters. One of his earliest memories is watching CNN's coverage of hurricanes and tornado aftermaths. Joshua's mind would race with lifesaving questions. "What would I do in that situation? Where would I hide? Where would I run?" he would ask himself.

Joshua didn't only find comfort in the safety of home; he also found it in food. "Food was my best friend growing up," he says. "We spent time together after school. We watched Saturday morning cartoons together and consoled each other when things got too difficult. Food never talked back to me, it never said an unkind word, and never let me down. The best part is it could change from ice cream to nachos to soda to leftovers depending on how I felt. It was a lifelong friend." His weight ballooned.

After graduating from high school, Joshua left Utah for 2 years to serve a Latter Day Saints mission in Chicago. "Quickly, I was thrown out of every comfort zone I ever knew," he says. "There was no going home for safety." Throughout his mission, he learned to embrace the anxiety, doubt, and uncertainty of standing outside of his comfort zone. He started taking control of his health. Within a year, he had lost nearly 60 pounds. Things were looking brighter.

When the mission in Chicago ended, he returned to Utah and enrolled in a local community college. But he felt depressed, and the weight he had lost came back. Over his 6 years of college, he started consulting other means of happiness, which most often included TV and a pizza. Sometimes even a bag of burgers.

When Joshua was 27 years old, he was diagnosed with hypothyroidism. Your thyroid gland sits below your Adam's apple in your neck. It synthesizes thyroid hormone, which plays a number of roles, including increasing your metabolic rate. Joshua's thyroid gland was underactive and thus did not produce enough thyroid hormone. The result was a slowing metabolism and, as Joshua experienced, weight gain and depression. He currently takes an oral thyroid hormone to counteract the hypothyroidism, but he doesn't make excuses. "Although my weight gain was from undiagnosed hypothyroidism, it was also from me," he says. "I was just letting life pass me by and doing nothing about it."

◆ ◆ ◆ ◆ ◆

THE FUNDAMENTAL DETERMINANT of body weight is caloric balance—the number of calories you consume through eating and drinking minus the number of calories you expend through physical activity, digestion of food, and all of your other daily activities. You use calories all the time. Every time you contract a muscle, either voluntarily or involuntarily, you use calories. Your other organs—heart, kidneys, liver, pancreas, brain, and so on—also use calories to carry out their varied functions.

Hippocrates wrote that "eating alone will not keep a man well; he must also take exercise." I'm not sure if Hippocrates ran, but if he did, he would have discovered that running is the most effective exercise to keep a man (or a woman) well, especially when it comes to losing weight and keeping it off. There are three major reasons why:

1 **Running creates a great need for energy.** When you run, you lower your carbohydrate fuel tank, you cause slight microscopic tears in your muscle fibers from the strong muscle contractions, and you increase body temperature. As soon as you stop running, your body naturally wants to return these things to their pre-exercise state. So, following a workout, your body rushes to replenish glycogen, repair the microscopic muscle tears, lower body temperature, and synthesize new structural and functional proteins as your body adapts. Your body requires energy (calories) to accomplish all of these tasks. If you don't run or do any other exercise, there is never a drain on muscle glycogen, nor any muscle tissue to repair or build, nor any reason to make new proteins, so any calories you consume that are greater than your metabolic needs are stored as fat. If you don't want your calories to be stored as fat, you need to exercise. Research shows that the amount people run is closely linked to how much weight they lose. And the converse is also true: The more runners decrease the amount of running they do, the more weight they put on.

> **" RESEARCH SHOWS THAT THE AMOUNT PEOPLE RUN IS CLOSELY LINKED TO HOW MUCH WEIGHT THEY LOSE."**

One of these studies is from the National Runners' and Walkers' Health Studies, the world's largest and longest-running series of studies on the health benefits of running and walking. Scientists divided 41,582 female runners into groups based on their age and the number of miles they ran per week. Compared with those who ran less than 10 miles per week, those who averaged over 40 miles per week had a 10 percent lower body mass index (your weight divided by your squared height; the most common value used to determine obesity), 8 percent lower waist circumference, 7 percent lower hip circumference, and 4 percent lower

RUN YOUR FAT OFF

chest circumference. In every age group, the greater the number of miles run per week, the lower the body mass index and chest, waist, and hip circumferences.

In another study from the National Runners' and Walkers' Health Studies, the researchers charted the running habits and body weight of 270 men and 146 women who started running, 3,973 men and 1,444 women who quit running, and 420 men and 153 women who remained sedentary during 7.5 years. They found that body weight and abdominal fat decreased in the people who started running and increased in the people who stopped running and in those who remained sedentary, with the changes proportional to the change in the amount they ran. In other words, the more the previously sedentary people ran, the greater the decrease in body weight and abdominal fat. Conversely, the more the runners reduced the amount they ran, the more their body weight and abdominal fat increased. Any runner who has ever been injured and can't run knows how easy and quick it is to put on weight. Running is one of the best ways to keep the weight off and become a leaner and fitter you.

2 **Running uses many muscles.** All the muscles in your legs (quadriceps, hamstrings, hip flexors, abductors, adductors, glutes, calves, and the muscles in the front of your shin) are used at different points in the running stride. You even use your abdominal muscles and the muscles in your shoulders a lot when you swing your arms back and forth as you run. The more muscles you use, the more oxygen you use, and the more oxygen you use, the more calories you burn.

3 **Running is weight bearing, which provides stress to the skeleton.** Every time your foot lands on the ground, your leg absorbs two to three times your body weight. Multiply that number by the number of steps you take on an average run, and multiply *that* by how many times you run each week, and you can see how much stress your legs have to deal with, especially if you're overweight. Because it threatens your body's survival to have all that stress on it, your body will do what it needs to do—shed weight—to alleviate the stress and assuage the threat to protect itself.

Can you burn calories, sculpt your butt and legs, and lose weight in ways other than running? Of course you can. But running burns and sculpts more. And that matters. Other forms of exercise burn so few calories that it's too easy to get the calories right back after completing a workout—the 30 minutes of walking or cycling it takes to burn 200 calories can be negated in just a few seconds with a glass of Gatorade and a handful of pretzels. Running, with its huge calorie burn, is your best chance to create an environment for fast weight loss and sculpt your lower body. The muscular forces generated when you run are nothing short of extraordinary. Because other activities don't use as many muscles and are not as weight bearing as running, you don't lose weight as quickly. These three principles are a central theme throughout this book and will guide you throughout your running and weight-loss journey.

HOW TO BURN MORE CALORIES WHEN RUNNING

You can estimate how many calories you burn when you run, which enables you to run smarter to lose weight. I'm sure you already know your current body weight and you'll know the duration of your run, of course. Next, you need to factor in your fitness level (represented by your maximum aerobic power, or VO_2max) and intensity (represented by the average percentage of your VO_2max during your run). Here's the equation you'll need:

Percent of VO_2max x VO_2max x Time x Weight x 5 calories per liter of O_2 consumed = **calories burned**

Let's take the example of a 180-pound female with a VO_2max that's average for her age. Here are her numbers:

1. Percent of VO_2max averaged during the run = **70 percent** (you can estimate this based on your percent of maximum heart rate)

2. VO_2max = **35 milliliters of oxygen per kilogram of body weight per minute**

3. Time spent running = **30 minutes**

4. Body weight = **180 pounds** (82 kilograms)

5. Number of calories used per liter (1,000 ml) of oxygen consumed = **5 calories** (this is a fixed number)

Now, plug these numbers into the equation and do some math:

$$0.70 \times \frac{35 \text{ ml}}{\text{kg/min}} \times 30 \text{ min} \times 82 \text{ kg} \times \frac{5 \text{ cal}}{1,000 \text{ ml } O_2} = \textbf{301 calories}$$

So, what does this tell us? In a 30-minute run, during which she's running at 70 percent of her VO_2max (which is a relatively comfortable pace, approximately 70 percent maximum heart rate), this woman burns about 300 calories. If she repeats this run three times per week, she'll burn 900 calories per week. If she also cuts 300 calories from her day, she'll have a weekly caloric deficit of 3,000 calories (300 calories × 7 days = 2,100 calories + 900 calories burned from running = 3,000 calories). At this rate, she'll lose about 0.85 pound per week (3,000 calories ÷ 3,500 calories per pound).

The equation also tells us how to burn more calories from running. Starting from the left side of the above equation, you could:

1. Run at a higher percentage of VO_2max
2. Increase VO_2max
3. Increase the amount of time spent running
4. Increase body weight

Although it's true that heavier people burn more calories when they run, your goal is to lose weight, not gain it, so obviously you can ignore the last option. The first option—run at a higher percentage of VO_2max—can work, but that, too, is not really practical. Running at a higher intensity (defined as running at a higher percent of your VO_2max) will decrease the amount of time you can run; the faster you run, the shorter the time you can hold the faster pace. (The easiest way to increase intensity is to run faster. But running uphill can also increase the intensity.) That leaves us with the second and third options—increasing your VO_2max and/or increasing the amount of time spent running. Both are effective for increasing the number of calories burned, but the second method—increasing your VO_2max—is the most effective and efficient. It enables you to burn more calories in the same amount of time. It also enables you to be more physically active because you are more aerobically fit. If our 180-pound woman from the above example increased her VO_2max from 35 to 45 and did the same 30-minute run at the same relative intensity (70 percent of VO_2max), she would burn 387 calories. If you use a combination of those two options—increasing your VO_2max *and* increasing the amount of time you spend running—you will burn even more calories.

Once you know how many calories you burn on your runs, you can determine how many calories you can eat and still meet your weight-loss goal. You can also use the above calculation the other way around—to determine how much and at what intensity you need to run to burn off the calories you eat.

How do you know what your VO_2max is? You can get it tested in a hospital or independent laboratory or volunteer to be part of a research study at a university, or you can use your maximum heart rate as a proxy for your VO_2max (see box below). Alternatively, although the exact number depends on your body weight and the amount of oxygen you consume to run at a given pace, research studies have estimated that you burn about 110 calories per mile run.

Now, you probably didn't pick up this book because you want to do math. You just want to run and lose weight. And you can. Just follow the running "menus" in Chapter 4 and eat a little bit less each day, and you will lose weight. But if you have a lot of weight to lose, you're going to have to get more serious about it.

HOW TO DETERMINE YOUR MAXIMUM HEART RATE

To determine your maximum heart rate, run 1 mile on a track or treadmill or other controlled environment while wearing a heart rate monitor. Start at a comfortable pace and pick up the pace every couple of minutes until you're running as fast as you can over the final couple of minutes. Check your heart rate monitor a few times over the final minute. The highest number you see is your maximum heart rate.

Your maximum aerobic power, or VO_2max, occurs when you are at your maximum heart rate, so maximum heart rate can be used as its proxy.

That means you will have to do a little figuring to determine how many calories you should eat and how much you should burn. And you'll need to monitor at least some of the calories coming in and going out. If you don't, you will most likely be eating more and burning fewer calories than you think. That prevents your waistline from getting slimmer.

So let's get started. I'm going to ask you to do something right now. Stop reading this, put the book down, and go run for 10 minutes (more if you can). If you need to mix walking and running, then do that. It doesn't matter how you run, what pace you run, or how much you run right now; you have to have a starting point. And there's no better time than right now to start it. So go. Right now. I'm not kidding. Go. I'll be here when you get back.

WHICH IS BETTER FOR WEIGHT LOSS:
Long, Slow Running or
High-Intensity Running?

Most proponents of high-intensity exercise come from a personal training or group fitness background. They tout the benefits of short, high-intensity workouts as a way to get fit and lose weight in less time. But the fitness and weight-loss industry often exaggerates things, including the amount that your metabolic rate increases following a workout. Metabolism does indeed increase after a high-intensity workout, so you will burn some calories after the workout is over, but it's the calories burned *during* the workout that matter more.

On the other hand, most proponents of long, slow running come from an endurance coaching background. They recognize that becoming a better runner requires a lot of aerobic running, and that weekly mileage has the single greatest impact on a runner's performance. And when you focus on performance, great things happen to the rest of your body.

Having a background in personal training, endurance coaching, *and* research science has given me a unique perspective. Truth is, you can burn lots of calories by running either long and slow or short and fast. Compared to other forms of exercise, even low-intensity running is relatively high intensity. In other words, even when you run slowly, you will get your heart rate and oxygen consumption up to 70 to 75 percent of their maximum. By contrast, if you were to ride a stationary bike in the gym or exercise to a workout DVD at home, you'd have to work pretty hard to get your heart rate and oxygen consumption that high. Pushing your running pace just a little can easily raise your heart rate and oxygen consumption to 85 to 90 percent of their maximum. I have yet to see a workout DVD you can do in your living room that will sustain your heart rate and oxygen consumption at 90 percent of their maximum.

High-intensity interval training is the most time-efficient way to burn calories and get fit. Fitness is important, because the fitter you become, the faster you can run. The faster you can run, the more distance you'll cover in a given amount of time. The more distance you cover in a given amount of time, the more calories you can burn in that time. Also, the fitter you become, the more physical work you can tolerate. I'd go so far to say that running interval workouts is the most effective type of exercise you can do to improve fitness and strengthen your cardiovascular system. It increases your heart rate and places a demand on your cardiovascular system in a way that nothing else does. And, given how busy everyone is, it pays to be time efficient.

> "HIGH-INTENSITY INTERVAL TRAINING IS THE MOST TIME-EFFICIENT WAY TO BURN CALORIES AND GET FIT."

On the surface, then, it seems that high-intensity running is better for weight loss, and it *can* be. However, over the long term, a high-volume, low-intensity approach is actually a more effective way to shed body fat. Even though high-intensity workouts burn more calories than do low-intensity workouts in the same amount of time, because of their high intensity, they are much shorter and you can do fewer of them. For example, if we use the sample person described earlier in this chapter with a VO_2max of 35 milliliters of oxygen per kilogram of body weight per minute, we can compare the number of calories burned between two different running workouts—a moderate-intensity run and a high-intensity interval workout. For reference, each calculation below is set up like the one on page 7: percent VO_2max

times VO$_2$max times the number of minutes spent running times body weight times the caloric cost of O$_2$ consumed:

Moderate-Intensity Run: 40 minutes at 70% VO$_2$max

$$0.70 \times \frac{35\ ml}{kg/min} \times 40\ min \times 82\ kg \times \frac{5\ cal}{1{,}000\ ml\ O_2} = \textbf{402 calories}$$

High-Intensity Interval Workout: Five 1-minute reps at 90% VO$_2$max with 2-minute jog recovery intervals between reps at 50% VO$_2$max (plus warm-up and cool-down)

Running reps portion:

$$0.90 \times \frac{35\ ml}{kg/min} \times 5\ min \times 82\ kg \times \frac{5\ cal}{1{,}000\ ml\ O_2} = \textbf{65 calories}$$

Jogging recovery intervals portion:

$$0.50 \times \frac{35\ ml}{kg/min} \times 8\ min \times 82\ kg \times \frac{5\ cal}{1{,}000\ ml\ O_2} = \textbf{57 calories}$$

Warm-up and cool-down portions:

$$0.60 \times \frac{35\ ml}{kg/min} \times 15\ min \times 82\ kg \times \frac{5\ cal}{1{,}000\ ml\ O_2} = \textbf{129 calories}$$

Total = 251 calories

Thus, in this example, the moderate-intensity run burns 151 more calories than the high-intensity interval workout (402 vs. 251). Even if we adjust the time of the moderate-intensity run to

28 minutes so the two workouts are the same amount of time, the moderate-intensity run still burns more calories (281) than the high-intensity workout. For the high-intensity workout to burn more calories, you would have to spend more time at the high intensity.

Realistically, you physically can't do an interval workout longer than about 15 minutes unless you are very fit, and you probably can't do more than two of these workouts per week, especially when you're a beginner. However, you can run slowly as long as you want and as often as you want—even every day if you have the time. So, over the course of a week, you can burn a lot more calories with long, slow runs than you can with interval workouts.

What if you *were* able to do enough high-intensity running to burn the equivalent number of calories as low-intensity running over the course of the week? Would you be able to lose more body weight and body fat? In this case, the research is mixed. A few studies show that high-intensity exercise is more effective at reducing body weight and body fat, while many more studies show no difference among varying exercise intensities. Taking all of the research together, it appears that for weight loss, it's the total number of calories burned, not the intensity of exercise, that matters.

Also, it is much easier for people to run long and slow than it is for them to run short and fast. High-intensity running is physically uncomfortable and, while that can be a good thing, people tend to shy away from what is physically uncomfortable. Every time I go to the track to do an interval workout, I'm the only one there. But when I go for easy runs around my neighborhood, I see many people doing the same thing. And if you walk into a gym and watch how people run on treadmills, nearly all of them are running at a slow pace while they either listen to music through their iPods or watch television on the TV monitors; hardly anyone is doing a high-intensity interval workout, focusing their attention on the hard effort. The explosion in popularity of the marathon and half marathon races in the United States and around the world attests to the same thing: People like running long, perhaps because humans have an innate interest in endurance. Humans like to push the limits of endurance, perhaps because when you push the limits of your own endurance, you find out how much you can endure. And that is a metaphor for life. Your ability to endure tough situations, your ability to endure poor health, your ability to endure stress—that is what makes you human.

So, the answer to the question "Which is better: long, slow running or high-intensity running?" is a bit complicated. It depends on what you're willing to do to get results and what you find more enjoyable so that you keep running for the rest of your life. The best strategy is to do both, or rather, to do all—to vary your workouts and run with the whole continuum of speeds, from very slow to very fast.

Variation is an important concept in exercise and fitness. Plenty of research has demonstrated that exercise programs with variation produce better results than those with no variation. When you vary the duration, volume, and intensity of your running, your body never has a chance to become efficient; it is always being challenged, always being forced to adapt. The trick to variation is knowing how and when to use it, because variation must be balanced with mastery of the skill. On one hand, you must repeat the same workout a number of times to master the volume and intensity so you can move forward with your running program, while on the other hand, you must vary your workouts often enough to avoid becoming too economical, improve your fitness, and lose weight.

One thing that holds beginner runners back is the intimidation of running fast and the discomfort they experience. A low-pressure, nonintimidating way to introduce faster-paced running is *fartlek,* a Swedish word meaning speedplay that returns us to running like we did as kids. Fartlek running dates back to 1937, when it was developed by Swedish coach Gösta Holmér, who used

RUNNING WITH OTHERS

Although running by yourself has its perks and gives you a chance—maybe the only one you have all day—to be alone, it helps to run with other people when you're trying to lose weight. Humans are social animals. Despite my introverted nature, every time I run with someone, I'm happy I did so. People can be a source of encouragement, inspiration, motivation, emotional support, laughter, and stories. And you'll need all of those when you're trying to lose weight.

And running with others holds you accountable. There's little doubt that running with others will help you stay on track with your new running habit. It's easier to push yourself when someone is running right next to you, even if neither of you says a word. A personal trainer or running coach will monitor what you do and help you modify your workouts to be most effective for you. Or, if you have a friend or two who want to lose weight, you can run with them.

There are also plenty of running groups all over the world with all different levels of runners that you can join, from small, informal groups to large, competitive, fee-based clubs that meet at a track for coach-led

it as part of Sweden's military training. During fartlek runs, you literally play with speed, picking up the pace at different times, when you reach specific landmarks, or just based on how you feel. Distances, speeds, and recovery periods all vary within the same workout.

formal workouts. There's even the unique Hash House Harriers, the self-proclaimed "drinking group with a running problem," who drink beer during their run. (You might want to stay away from that group if you're trying to lose weight.)

The easiest way to find a running group is to Google "running clubs" and your city and state. For a more specific search, add terms like "recreational" or "weight loss." If you're interested in an informal group, there are hundreds of local running groups around the country, most of which meet on a regular basis for runs of varying distances based on people's abilities. Many running shoe stores also lead informal groups that meet in front of their stores for weekly evening runs.

Perhaps, most of all, running with others gives you a chance to share—to share your highs, your lows, your funny stories, your passions, your experiences of being runners, and your weight-loss journeys. Gaining strength from that of others, witnessing their passion, seeing how they overcome difficulties in their lives can help bring out the best in you.

◆ ◆ ◆ ◆ ◆

"I TOOK BABY STEPS," says Joshua Snow Hansen, who, at 218 pounds, is half the person he used to be when he weighed 402 pounds. "I didn't jump right into a hardcore weight-loss program; I just changed habits. I watched what I ate, walked more, and drank more water than soda. Within the first month of just doing that, I lost about 30 pounds. That success fueled me to try harder."

Joshua's running journey started with a 5K. "My friend Kevin, a personal trainer, helped me overcome a lot of my fears of the gym and taught me how to use the gym to get the most out of it. I began to see big physical changes. Soon I was down 50 pounds, 75 pounds, and then 100 pounds. After losing close to 100 pounds, Kevin challenged me to start training for a 5K.

"On the morning of the 5K, I was nervous. I honestly didn't have the right equipment. My shoes were a couple years old and my gym shorts were bought at the peak of my weight. If it wasn't for a good elastic band, I probably would have lost my shorts mid-run. But I was prepared and I had to put trust into my training and Kevin's instruction.

"I won't say it was love at first run," Joshua says. "It was a process. I felt like I was running uphill both ways. My legs hurt and my lungs struggled to keep up, but I was running alongside Kevin and he kept me going. As exhausted and tired as I felt at the finish line, this odd feeling swept over me. I wanted more."

A month later, he signed up for his second 5K, then another, and another. "The thing I love about running," he says, "is that your success is based on your effort. Your best is always right in front of you." He then found the courage to train for a 10K. His stamina and strength grew, and he continued to lose weight. "Soon, I found myself down 125 pounds, 150 pounds, and, within 3$\frac{1}{2}$ years, 180 pounds. Running was changing my life."

And the races kept getting longer. Shortly before we spoke, Joshua ran his first ultramarathon (any race longer than a standard 26.2-mile marathon). "I had no ambition to be running half, full, or ultramarathons," he says. "I just wanted to do better at another 5K. But that challenge led me to run a 10K, then a half marathon, then a full marathon, and then an ultramarathon."

He set a long-term goal to run 180 races of a half marathon or longer before his 40th birthday. Rather ambitious for a guy in his late 20s who just started running. "Six years ago, I would have never imagined being *here*," he says, emphasizing that last word as if running has literally brought him to a different place. "I would have never imagined myself being a runner, especially an ultramarathoner.

"The choice to begin running was simple," he says. "I decided I had enough. I wasn't living the life I wanted or dreamed about." At his college graduation, he could barely fit into his graduation gown. "When I sat down, I ripped my gown," he says. "After faking smiles for pictures, I had a lot of time that night to think about the day's events. I knew that my feelings needed to be addressed. I didn't have a vision of the future, and it didn't help that I busted the crotch out of my graduation gown. I was growing even sicker of the person that I was, and I knew that I had to wake up and begin living life. So I started waking up."

I realized that Joshua had just revealed to me the *real* secret to lasting weight loss: Don't go on a diet or take up running to lose weight. Make the decision to be happier and live a more fulfilling life. That decision will direct your efforts. When you strive toward a goal and to become a better version of yourself, the weight will come off. "When I made the decision to be happier and live a more fulfilling life, the weight was the easiest place to start," he says.

Joshua is pretty routine in his daily approach to his runs, meals, and other habits. Instead of throwing something in the office mailbox at work, he hand-delivers the mail. Instead of sitting at his desk watching Netflix during lunch, he takes a walk. And he keeps that behavior consistent. "Once I lost 100 to 150 pounds, I realized just how important consistency was in my journey," he says. But things haven't always been easy. Joshua's weight still fluctuates from the hypothyroidism. "If running has taught me anything, it has taught me to fight through the downs instead of being complacent."

When asked what advice he has for others, he says, "It doesn't matter what your size, experience, or fitness level is; just get out and run. No one cares how you look running, because everyone looks ridiculous running. Have you ever looked through race photos? Don't worry about it. Be out on the road or trail for the right reasons. For you.

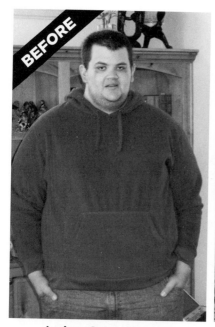

Joshua Snow Hansen at 402 pounds.

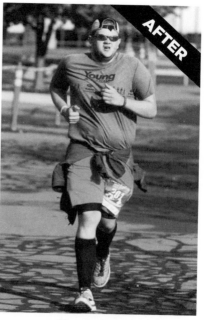

Hansen now, at 218 pounds.

"And don't go about your journey alone. Join a club, find a Facebook running club, or grab a friend you want to go on the journey with. You will have more success sticking to your diet and training plan if you involve yourself with the community and hold yourself accountable through other people."

I couldn't end our conversation without asking him about that goal of running 180 races before his 40th birthday. Why 180? "I chose 180 races as my goal for many reasons," he says. "One, because I lost 180 pounds; two, because it's the name of my blog, Running180.com; and three, because running has turned my life around 180 degrees."

After being away on his mission and transferring from community college to a university 3 hours away, Joshua decided to go back home. This time, he's running back.

CHAPTER 2

Calories and Metabolism

"I USED TO BE THE GIRL WHO CLAIMED THAT 'I DON'T RUN UNLESS I'M BEING CHASED.'"

EXIT **124** OFF THE GARDEN STATE PARKWAY puts you in the suburban town of Sayreville, located on the Raritan River in New Jersey's Middlesex County, just 36 miles southwest of New York's Times Square. When I spoke with Sayreville resident Jessica Skarzynski, who grew up in nearby South Amboy, she was getting ready to run her seventh half marathon. This was a big deal for her because she was always overweight and was never athletic.

At 21 years old, she reached her heaviest weight of 275 pounds. "I was in college and building an awesome new path in life for myself, but I didn't feel skinny enough to do the things that other people around me were doing," she says. "I didn't want to date or go out to nightclubs and bars because I was afraid of what others would think of me. I took every whisper, every look, every dating rejection as a result of my weight and my appearance, so I put up a wall." By 2004, a serious anxiety disorder crippled her emotionally and physically. The only medication that helped also started cravings that packed on the pounds.

A few days before her twenty-first birthday, her mother was diagnosed with breast cancer. Jessica was crushed. "After breaking down in the hallway of our house, I decided to go to the park later that day to run myself into oblivion. I had never run more than a mile, but I needed to numb the pain and couldn't think of anything else to do. So I ran. I didn't care about what *anyone* thought of me that day."

We all have our tipping point, that event or circumstance or moment that makes us act, that makes us do something we wouldn't otherwise do. For Jessica, the tipping point was her mom's cancer diagnosis.

Jessica learned how to listen to her body and eat sensibly. She started slowly at first—a half hour on the stationary bike in her college dorm's gym a few times per week and smarter choices in the dining hall. "After burning myself out on my run in the park, I started to pay closer attention to my choices—what I ate, how I moved, how I spent my free time," she says. In 1 year, she dropped 40 pounds. "I found myself addicted to the high of working out, and when I started running, I really discovered my happy place," she says. But that was only just the beginning.

◆ ◆ ◆ ◆ ◆

DESPITE WHAT MOST PEOPLE, and especially those celebrity trainers trying to sell their newest fad diets, want to believe, our genes actually play a large role in determining how much we weigh. Our genetic code contains the blueprint for our body type. Our environment only plays a role in obesity in that it enables those obesogenic genes to be expressed.

Take, for example, a study from Denmark, in which the researchers compared the weight of more than 500 adopted children with that of their biological parents and that of their adoptive parents. If learned eating habits influence a child's body weight more than genes do, his or her body weight should be similar to his or her adoptive parents. Conversely, if genes influence a child's body weight more than environment does, his or her body weight should be similar to that of the biological parents. What did the researchers find? Interestingly, the children's body weight was highly correlated with the weight of their biological parents but not with the weight of their adoptive parents, even though their biological parents were not raising them.

Another great way to test the gene theory of body weight is to study identical twins. In the Swedish Adoption/Twin Study of Aging, researchers compared the body weight of 93 pairs of identical twins who were raised apart in separate homes and 154 pairs of identical twins raised together in the same home. The results of the study showed that the body weights of the identical twins were highly correlated whether the twins were raised together or apart. The results of this and other twin studies have shown that genes account for 70 percent of the variation in people's body weight. That's a pretty large influence.

YOUR SET POINT

Based on your genes, your brain has its own sense of what you should weigh, no matter what you consciously believe. This is called your *set point,* which is really a set weight range of about 10 to 15 pounds. Your brain—not your willpower nor your conscious decisions—responds to weight loss by using powerful tools to push your weight back up to what it considers normal. If you lose a lot of weight, your brain reacts as if it were starving, and your body will burn less energy during the day because resting metabolism decreases when you lose weight. Although this was a successful survival strategy to conserve energy during the time of our early ancestors when food was scarce, it is not a good strategy in our obesogenic environment where high-caloric foods are in overabundance. This means that a successful weight loser—someone who does not gain the weight back—must forever eat fewer calories than someone of the same weight who has always been that weight.

This doesn't mean that you don't have any control over how much you weigh. Of course you do, as evidenced by reality TV shows such as *The Biggest Loser*. Genes may account for 70 percent of the variation in weight, but the other 30 percent is up to you. Your choices still matter. Your willpower matters. You may not choose to be fat, but you do choose to be thin. The people whose stories are woven through this book are proof that you do have control over your weight and many aspects of your health. It's not a coincidence that two-thirds of the U.S. adult population is overweight or obese, and less than one-fifth of the population exercises on a regular basis. Behavior matters.

METABOLISM

Metabolism is one of those buzzwords that people often talk about but don't really understand. Pick up any fitness or weight-loss book at your local bookstore and the word *metabolism* is all over the pages. Hollywood personal trainers and celebrity authors are quick to act like they are metabolism experts and say a lot of things about metabolism that, at the very least, show a rudimentary understanding and, at worst, are not true. What is metabolism, really, and how does running affect it?

Metabolism is the sum of all chemical reactions in living cells by which energy is provided for vital life processes. It is the amount of energy (calories) required each day to keep your body functioning—the energy that keeps your heart beating, your brain thinking, your lungs breathing, and many other cellular processes occurring.

In 1780, Frenchmen Antoine Laurent Lavoisier and Pierre-Simon

Laplace were the first scientists to study and quantify metabolism. By measuring how much oxygen guinea pigs consumed and how much carbon dioxide they produced while sitting in a *calorimeter* (a device for measuring heat energy that is sealed off to the outside environment) doing normal guinea pig things, Lavoisier and Laplace could calculate the metabolic rate—how many calories the guinea pig used. Pretty ingenious, huh?

The processes that control and affect metabolism are an enormously complex subject that includes the interdisciplinary fields of biology, physiology, chemistry, and physics. Adding the conditions of food intake and exercise makes the understanding of metabolism even more complex. For example, when Lavoisier and chemist Armand Séguin studied the influence of food intake and muscular work on metabolism, they discovered that resting energy metabolism increased by 50 percent due to food intake, 200 percent due to exercise, and 300 percent by combining food intake with exercise.

Your resting metabolic rate—how much energy your body needs to live—makes up about 60 to 75 percent of your daily energy expenditure. It has been set from millions of years of evolution. It is a relatively stable, constrained physiological trait for the human species, more a product of our common genetic inheritance than our diverse lifestyles. All humans require a certain amount of metabolic activity for their bodies to function normally. Because all humans operate at nearly identical temperatures and human organs are standard (your healthy liver is nearly identical to my healthy liver), all humans have a nearly identical resting metabolism once body size and body composition are accounted for.

Resting metabolic rate, which is typically measured as the amount of oxygen you consume at rest relative to your body weight, averages 3.5 milliliters of oxygen per kilogram of body weight per minute. For every liter (1,000 milliliters) of oxygen you consume, you burn 5 calories. Therefore, at rest, humans burn about 0.0175 calorie per kilogram of body weight per minute (3.5 × 5 ÷ 1,000). For a 150-pound (68-kilogram) person, that's 1.19 calories per minute, or 1,714 calories per day. For a 200-pound (91-kilogram) person, that's 1.59 calories per minute, or 2,290 calories per day. Thus, a heavier person has a greater resting metabolic rate than does a lighter person and will burn more calories per day.

Resting metabolism is also affected by age and sex, but only by how much muscle is affected by age and sex. Men have a slightly faster metabolism not because they are men, but because they typically have more muscle mass. The same is true for age—metabolism slows with age not because of age *per se*, rather because of the loss of muscle mass that typically accompanies aging. You can't do much to boost your resting metabolic rate, but you can increase your muscle mass—and thus keep your resting metabolic rate from slowing down—with resistance training. Muscle burns more calories than fat per pound, even at rest. Muscle also looks much better on your body and is easier to carry around and run with. Fat is just extra weight that sits there like an annoying in-law who won't leave.

HOW RUNNING AFFECTS METABOLISM

While your resting metabolic rate is relatively constrained, you *can* increase your active metabolic rate. When you run, your metabolic rate increases dramatically from what it is when you're sitting on the couch reading this book. The best runners in the world, who consume oxygen at very high rates when running fast, can increase their metabolic rate 25 times its resting value. A person of average to above-average fitness can increase his or her metabolic rate about 10 to 15 times from what it is at rest. That's why running is so effective at burning calories quickly—because of its ability to raise your metabolic rate to a level much higher than when you're sitting at your desk or at your dining room table, and much higher than other types of exercise because of its greater use of muscle mass and because of the demand created by bearing two to three times your body weight.

The faster you run, the more your metabolic rate increases, in part because your muscles increase their demand for oxygen so they can continue to maintain the speed. In response to this increased demand for oxygen, your heart rate and stroke volume (the volume of blood your heart pumps with each beat) both increase to send more blood and oxygen to your muscles. Also, the vessels just below your skin dilate and more blood is sent to your skin to increase your ability to cool yourself as your body temperature rises. And your diaphragm and other breathing muscles work harder since you breathe heavier to exhale the carbon dioxide that starts to build up in your blood from the increased intensity of your run. These are all energy-requiring processes, which collectively raise your metabolic rate while you run. Your metabolic rate remains elevated for a while after your run as muscle glycogen (the stored form of carbohydrate) is replaced and your body repairs itself and builds the structures that your run has stimulated to be built. Therefore, one way to increase how many calories you burn when you run is to expand your body's capacity to consume oxygen. How do you do that? You run more and you run faster.

CARBOHYDRATE VERSUS FAT METABOLISM

When you run, you use a combination of two fuels—fat and carbohydrate—to supply energy for all of the energy-requiring processes. Protein, the third major macronutrient, accounts for only about 5 to 10 percent of energy production during exercise and so is usually neglected as a fuel. Rather, proteins are primarily used in building, maintaining, and repairing muscle, skin, and blood tissue, and aid in the transportation of materials through the blood. However, the body's requirement for energy takes priority over tissue building, so protein can be used as an energy source if your muscles don't have an adequate amount of fat and carbohydrate (like in the case of low-carb diets).

You store fat in three places—directly beneath your skin (adipose tissue), within your muscles (intramuscular triglycerides), and around your abdominal organs (visceral fat). Humans' store of adipose fat (the fat that you see on your hips, thighs, and belly) is virtually unlimited, even in very thin people. Even a 145-pound person with 18 percent body fat has enough fat fuel to last about 5 days of long-distance running or about 1,000 miles of walking. While people would love to see their bellies shrink while running on the treadmill or through the park, most of the fat you use when you run is of the intramuscular triglyceride variety because the fat stored inside your muscles is physically closer to where it is ultimately used for energy and so is therefore more efficient to use. It's during the rest of the day, when you are not running, that fat is lost from the adipose tissue on your left butt cheek and other places where fat is stored.

Although adipose fat gets all the attention, visceral fat—the fat you can't see that surrounds your abdominal organs—is even more important. Too much visceral fat has huge implications for your health, including impaired glucose and fat metabolism; insulin resistance; increased predisposition to colon, breast, and prostate cancer; prolonged hospital stays and increased mortality in the hospital; increased incidence of infections and noninfectious complications; incidence of metabolic syndrome; and increased susceptibility to heart disease and high blood pressure. Visceral fat is a bad, bad thing. Research has shown that aerobic exercise is central to reduce visceral fat.

You also store carbohydrate in two places—in your blood as the sugar glucose and in your skeletal muscles and liver as glycogen. You use both of these sources of carbohydrate when you run. Unlike your unlimited store of fat, you have enough stored carbohydrate in your muscles and liver to provide enough energy for only about 100 minutes of sustained running at a moderate pace. At slow running speeds, some of carbohydrate's metabolic responsibility for energy production is relieved by fat, in the form of free fatty acids in the blood and intramuscular triglyceride. Even with the contribution of fat helping to delay the depletion of glycogen, you can sustain a moderate pace for only 2 to 3 hours.

If you run for a prolonged period of time (more than 2 hours), blood glucose gets very low and your muscles and liver can also run low on glycogen. When this happens, fat metabolism predominates, with adipose tissue releasing large quantities of fatty acids into the blood so they can travel to the muscles and be used for energy (in addition to the increased reliance on intramuscular triglycerides). Some people recommend running in a glycogen-depleted state, like first thing in the morning before breakfast, in order to force a greater use of fat. But fat burns in a carbohydrate flame. When you force your body to burn fat without adequate carbohydrate present, the products of fat metabolism form ketones in the liver, causing a condition known as *ketosis*. This causes your blood to become acidic and can cause you to feel shaky, fatigued, or dizzy, which impairs your ability to run. The depletion of glycogen also causes an increase in amino acid (protein) metabolism and an associated increase in blood and muscle ammonia, which can be toxic to muscle cells. Have you ever smelled the breath of someone who has been exercising on a low-carb diet? That's the smell of ammonia. So, don't run when you are glycogen depleted.

Carbohydrate, not fat, is muscles' preferred fuel during exercise. Carbohydrate is muscles' chocolate—they prefer to consume it over everything else. That's why it's such a threat to our health when we run out of it. Not only does low blood glucose and glycogen depletion lead to ketosis, it also compromises immune function. Although research has shown that diets low in carbohydrate can lead to short-term weight loss, they cannot be sustained permanently. For this reason, I do not recommend going on a low-carb diet for an extended period of time.

Although you use both fat and carbohydrate for energy when you run, these two fuels provide that energy on a sliding scale—as you increase your running pace, the contribution from fat decreases while the contribution from carbohydrate increases. The intensity and duration of the activity are the primary determinants of how much of each fuel you use. This is where people often make a critical mistake when it comes to fat burning. Because more fat is used at low intensities of exercise, it is often assumed that low-intensity exercise is best for burning fat. Even manufacturers of cardio equipment include "fat-burning" zones on their front panels that promote exercise at a low intensity. Although it's true that the slower you run, the more your muscles rely on fat compared to carbohydrate, the *rate* of energy use—the number of calories burned per minute—is low. At faster running speeds, both the *rate* of energy use and the *total number* of calories you expend are much greater, such that the absolute amount of fat used is also greater. Therefore, the rate of overall energy expenditure (i.e., the total number of calories you burn), rather than simply the percentage of energy derived from fat, is very important when it comes to fat loss. In other words, don't rely on low-intensity exercise alone to lose weight.

RUNNING AND FAT BURNING

Want to know a secret of losing fat? *You don't have to use fat when you run to lose fat from your waistline.* What? That doesn't make any sense. If I want to lose fat from my hips and thighs, shouldn't I be burning fat when I run? Not necessarily. Running significantly increases *lipolysis*—the breakdown of fat—by increasing activity of the enzyme lipoprotein lipase and decreases *lipogenesis*—the formation and subsequent storage of body fat. Conversely, inactivity suppresses lipoprotein lipase, thus inhibiting fat burning.

You can become lean and obtain a low percentage of body fat even if you run at a high intensity that uses carbohydrate for energy. Your body fat, which is the fat from adipose tissue underneath your skin, is lost during the hours *after* you finish your run. All of the things that your body has to do to recover and recreate balance after running require energy. Recovery itself requires energy. That energy comes from fat, and the amount of fat transported and used after your run depends, in part, on the intensity *during* the run. Following high-intensity running, more fat from adipose tissue is transported to the muscles, and muscles use fat at a faster rate.

> **" YOU DON'T HAVE TO USE FAT WHEN YOU RUN TO LOSE FAT FROM YOUR WAISTLINE."**

By tinkering with your running workouts, you can burn more calories both during and after your runs. As you become more fit, you recover faster, so your postworkout metabolic rate returns to its resting level sooner. Although some of the research comparing postworkout metabolic rates between trained and untrained people is a bit contradictory due to differences in research methods, most research has shown that postworkout metabolic rate is elevated longer in *untrained* people. (Out-of-shape people take longer to recover from a run.) Although the elevation in metabolism after your runs helps you burn more calories, the elevated metabolism *during* your workouts (which is much higher than afterward) has a greater impact on your calorie burn and subsequent weight loss.

CALORIES

To find out how many calories you need to expend to lose weight, we must travel back in time to 1958, when Dr. Max Wishnofsky concluded (based on previous research in 1930) that the caloric equivalent of 1 pound (0.45 kilogram) of body weight lost is approximately 3,500 calories. He also explained that as weight loss occurs, resting metabolic rate decreases. For example, if a 40-year-old, 5-foot-10, 300-pound male reduces his weight to 200 pounds, his resting metabolic rate would drop from 2,265 calories to 1,995 calories, a difference of 270 calories per day or 8,100 calories per month. Thus, if he continues on the same activity and diet program, he would lose 2.3 pounds less per month (8,100 ÷ 3,500) at 200 pounds compared to when he was 300 pounds. In other words, if he had started out by losing 8 pounds per month, he would now be losing 5.7 pounds per month.

People don't lose weight linearly over time, as Wishnofsky pointed out so many years ago. Weight loss is often dynamic rather than linear, and your body's energy requirements change as you lose weight and alter your body composition and metabolic rate. When resting metabolic rate decreases as you lose weight, you need less energy, so calorie restriction no longer has the same effect as it did at the beginning of your diet program. So, what does this mean? Initially, when you lose weight, you'll likely lose 1 pound (or very close to it) for every 3,500-calorie deficit you accumulate. However, as you lose a substantial amount of weight and your metabolic rate starts to drop, it will take more than 3,500 calories to lose 1 pound.

What the Heck Is a Calorie, Anyway?

In our society, there's a lot of commotion about calories. They're everywhere we turn—in the news, on food labels, in menus, on our plates, and in our glasses and cups. I swear they even hide under my bed. We are consumed, figuratively and literally, with calories.

When I was first taught in high school what a calorie is, I admit it took me a while to understand. But that's okay, because the world doesn't understand either, and that's why we have diet gurus proposing that mysterious concepts other than "calories in versus calories out" are responsible for weight loss.

A calorie is a measurement of energy. Specifically, it's the amount of heat energy needed to raise the temperature of 1 gram of water by 1 degree Celsius. That's kind of esoteric, unless you plan on heating a gram of water on your stove and measuring its energy. What's important to understand is that when we talk about calories, we are talking about energy. Despite the bad rap that calories get, a calorie is neither good nor bad. It just is.

Calories are used by nutritionists and dietitians to measure the amount of energy contained in the chemical bonds of the nutrients in food. Every food label includes the number of calories (energy) per serving (or, more precisely, the number of kilocalories, which equals 1,000 calories). That is, if a serving of bread has 100 calories, the nutrients in the bread contain enough heat energy to raise the temperature of 100 grams of water by one degree Celsius.

In terms of weight loss and weight gain, all calories are created equal—each calorie contains a specific amount of energy. There is no debating that; the definition of the calorie and the relationship between energy and matter, including muscle and fat, is subject to the laws of thermodynamics. To understand this, we must seek out the advice of someone much smarter than me: Albert

Einstein. Einstein's famous equation ($E = mc^2$) tells us that the energy of an object is equal to the mass of that object multiplied by the square of the speed of light. The speed of light, and thus its square, is a constant value and doesn't change (unless you change the medium in which the light travels, such as in water or outer space). Thus, the energy of an object is proportional to its mass. You change the amount of energy (calories) stored in that object, and you change the object's mass. Remember this, because we're going to come back to it later.

Every diet guru or celebrity health nut who claims that not all calories are created equal is going up against Einstein and the laws of thermodynamics. Debating whether a calorie is really a calorie is akin to debating whether gravity is really gravity. There are no different "kinds" of calories, just as there are no different "kinds" of gravity. In terms of energy consumption, it makes no difference whether a calorie is from a carrot or from carrot cake. The *quantity* of calories you consume matters; it's the principal determinant of what the scale reads when you stand on it.

Running is the best and fastest way to expend those calories, making it the best method for weight loss. Every mile you run burns about 110 calories (technically, kilocalories), give or take, depending on how much you weigh and your running economy (i.e., how much oxygen your body uses to run at a given pace). The more you weigh, the more calories you'll actually burn every mile or kilometer because it takes more oxygen and more energy to transport a heavier weight than it does to transport a lighter weight. (Try running with a loaded backpack; you'll quickly discover how much more energy that takes.)

Despite the claims written on the covers of many weight loss books and those made during late-night television infomercials, sustained weight loss occurs at a rate of $1/2$ to 2 pounds per week. It's simply a matter of math: To lose weight at a more rapid rate, you would have to severely cut back on the number of calories you consume and exercise all day long to achieve the caloric deficit you would need to lose weight faster. That doesn't mean you can't lose weight more rapidly than at the rate of $^1/_2$ to 2 pounds per week. But you have to be realistic. The rate at which you lose weight depends on a number of factors, not the least of which is how much you weigh to begin with. When you understand how large of a caloric deficit it takes to lose just 1 pound, it becomes clear why it's hard to lose weight at a faster rate. And losing weight at a faster rate does not give you any better chance of keeping it off.

" RUNNING IS THE BEST AND FASTEST WAY TO EXPEND THOSE CALORIES, MAKING IT THE BEST METHOD FOR WEIGHT LOSS.

For example, research from Maastricht University Medical Center in Maastricht, the Netherlands, published in the journal *Obesity,* has shown that when individuals consume a very low-calorie diet (500 calories per day), they lose weight rapidly (10 percent reduction in body weight in 5 weeks). However, the amount of weight regained is similar to when individuals lose weight more slowly (10 percent reduction in body weight in 12 weeks) on a low-calorie diet (1,250 calories per day). So it's possible to lose weight rapidly by consuming a very low-calorie diet, but how long do you think you can sustain a diet of just 500 calories per day? A much better strategy is to consume a low-calorie diet and to run because that is much more sustainable.

When you first start running, you'll initially burn a lot of calories because you're not very economical. As your body gets used to running, your economy improves—meaning you'll use less oxygen to run at a given pace. This is a good thing if you want to become a faster runner, but it's not so good if you want to burn as many calories as you can on each run. One way to minimize improvements in economy so you can burn more calories every mile or kilometer is to vary your runs. Don't run the same distance in the same place at the same pace every day. Instead, vary

> **" SUSTAINED WEIGHT LOSS OCCURS AT A RATE OF 1/2 TO 2 POUNDS PER WEEK."**

the speeds and distances and terrain of your runs. Some days run slowly, some days run fast, some days run long, some days run hills. The more varied your runs, the more calories you'll burn.

Where Do Calories Go?

Your muscles can't directly convert calories from the food you eat into the energy needed to move your body. As your high school biology teacher taught, the energy for movement comes from the chemical breakdown of a high-energy metabolic compound in your cells called *adenosine triphosphate* (ATP). ATP is your energy currency. When the strong chemical bonds of ATP are broken, heat and energy are liberated and muscles contract. The breakdown of ATP is necessary for every single movement you make, from blinking your eyes to running a marathon. Since your muscles don't store much ATP, you must constantly resynthesize it before breaking it down. The formation and resynthesis of ATP is thus a circular process—ATP is broken down into its constituents— adenosine diphosphate (ADP) and phosphate (P)—which then recombine to resynthesize ATP.

The calories contained in the carbohydrate, fat, and protein you eat and drink are used to synthesize ATP through many chemical reactions to meet cells' large need for energy to perform different tasks. But what if it's a slow day at the office and your cells don't need a lot of energy? What if you already have enough ATP lying around in your cells to meet their needs? When you consume carbohydrate, fat, and protein, where do the calories go?

A few years ago, I was standing in the diet and weight-loss book aisle of a bookstore, talking to a woman about losing weight. "I walk 2 miles a day 5 days a week and I'm still not losing weight," she told me, sounding frustrated. I tried to explain to her how many calories each mile of walking burns and the "calories out" part of the weight-loss equation. If I had had a pencil and piece of paper with me, I would have drawn her this diagram:

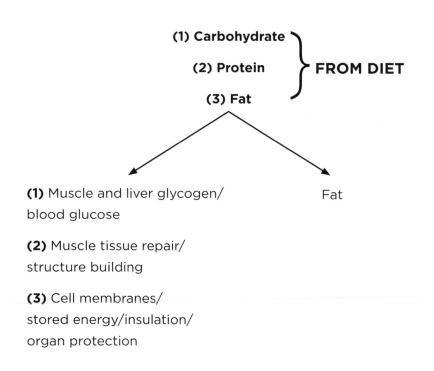

Following the left arrow in the diagram above and matching up the numbers, you can see what carbohydrate, fat, and protein are used for in your body. Carbohydrate is used for fuel by your muscles and exists in your body in two forms: glucose in your blood and glycogen (a branched chain of glucose molecules, which is the stored form of carbohydrate) in your muscles and liver. Any carbohydrate that you eat is used to replenish blood glucose and muscle and liver glycogen. Protein is used to build things like muscle tissue, enzymes, and other parts of cells that carry out specific functions. Fat is an important component of cell membranes and is used as a fuel, as insulation, and to protect your internal organs. Where things go awry is when you follow the right arrow in the diagram on page 39. If your body doesn't need to carry out the functions to the left, *all* of the extra calories from carbohydrate, fat, and protein follow the path of the right arrow and are stored as fat. You and the other 2.1 billion people in the world who are overweight are overweight because the calories you consume follow the path of the right arrow. It's as simple as that.

Your level of physical activity and your caloric intake are tightly coupled over a wide range of physical activities. However, this tight coupling is lost in people who don't exercise at all, and caloric intake is inappropriately high, which causes people to gain weight.

The big secret to not gaining weight is to never go down the path of the right arrow. How do you do that? You must create an environment that forces the calories to follow the left arrow. How do you create such an environment? I'm glad you asked.

HOW RUNNING AFFECTS WHERE CALORIES GO

Running lowers your carbohydrate fuel tank, which creates a metabolic demand because carbohydrate is the muscles' preferred fuel. Lowering that fuel tank is threatening to the survival of your muscles, so any carbohydrate you eat will be used to refill the tank. The synthesis and storage of glycogen—the refilling of the carbohydrate fuel tank—is controlled by the hormone insulin and the availability and uptake of glucose from the blood. Through its effect on specific proteins that transport glucose, insulin draws glucose from the blood into muscle cells to be stored. The glucose is then used to make new glycogen. The higher the blood insulin concentration and the greater the availability of glucose, the faster glycogen is synthesized and stored.

The same thing happens with protein. When you run, you send a signal to build structural and functional proteins and you cause microscopic damage to the muscle fibers, so the amino acids from any protein you eat will be used to build those structural and functional proteins and repair the damage to the muscle fibers to make them stronger and more durable.

To prevent fat from accumulating on those love handles, you must create a metabolic demand so that the calories are used for other, more important needs. Make the love handles wait. If you are always mobilizing energy for it to be used, you're not storing it as fat. Running creates the metabolic demands, giving you the director's clapperboard so that *you* decide where the calories go. And that is exactly one of the goals of the *Run Your Fat Off* program—to make *you* the director of the calorie movie, dictating where your calories go and how they are used.

WEIGHT MAINTENANCE

Once you lose weight, you want to keep it off. There is little point to going through the exercise (pun intended) of losing weight if you're just going to regain it. Maintaining lost weight is itself a lot of work, and most diets don't emphasize the critical aspect of being able to maintain weight.

Just as your body adapts to every running stride you take, so, too, does it adapt to the pounds you lose. A multitude of hormones are involved in the regulation of body weight, the concentrations of which are altered after you lose weight. Many of these alterations persist for at least a year after you start to lose weight, even after you have started to gain the weight back, suggesting that the high rate of weight regain among dieters has a strong physiological basis and is not simply the result of lack of willpower or the resumption of old habits.

Because most weight-loss studies are of short duration, the only reliable proof of what works for permanent weight loss comes from the people who have actually achieved permanent weight loss. And the studies that have examined those people have shown that no one diet is better than any other. Behavioral factors—monitoring weight, exercising daily—matter more.

For example, in a study by a group of scientists at the University of Colorado–Denver, the physical activity patterns of weight losers in the National Weight Control Registry were examined. Successful weight losers engaged in an average of 41.5 minutes per day (290 minutes per week) of sustained moderate-to-vigorous physical activity, while a control group of overweight individuals exercised an average of just 19.2 minutes per day (134 minutes per week) and a control group of normal-weight individuals exercised an average of 25.8 minutes per day (181 minutes per week).

In another study from the Brown University Medical School and Miriam Hospital in Providence, Rhode Island, scientists compared the amount and intensity of exercise of successful female weight losers to individuals who had never been overweight. To be in the study, the people in the weight-loss group had to have had a body mass index (BMI) of at least 25 at some point in their lives, but at the time of the study were of normal weight (with a BMI between 18.5 and 25), had lost at least 10 percent of their maximum body weight, and kept off at least 10 percent of their weight for at least 5 years. Conversely, the people in the always-normal-weight group had no history of being overweight or obese (defined as a BMI of at least 25) and had to have always had a BMI between 18.5 and 25. Their weight also had to be stable, being within 10 pounds of their weight for at least 2 years prior to the study. The scientists discovered that the weight-loss maintainers spent more total time being physically active and spent more time doing high-intensity exercise when compared to the always-normal-weight group.

What do we learn from this research? Individuals who have lost weight require more exercise to maintain their new weight and BMI than individuals who have never been overweight and who weigh the same and have a similar BMI as the previously overweight person. In other words, if you're 200 pounds and you lose 50 pounds so that you're now 150 pounds, you will always need more exercise to maintain your 150-pound weight than will your friend who has always been 150 pounds. But why? Why isn't 150 pounds always 150 pounds?

Energy balance, like most of human physiology, is largely regulated by your central nervous system, which senses metabolic status from a wide range of hormonal and neural signals and controls energy intake. In other words, when you're thin, your central nervous system "knows" you're thin because of the feedback it gets from specific hormones, and it regulates your appetite and storage of fat accordingly. When you're overweight, your central nervous system "knows" you're overweight because of the *different* feedback it gets from specific hormones, and it regulates your appetite and storage of fat accordingly. When you're overweight and *lose* weight, your central nervous system "thinks" it needs to "correct" for your weight loss and it activates multiple compensatory mechanisms (making you feel more hungry, for instance), including changes in circulating hormones and reductions in resting metabolic rate and the efficiency of your mitochondria to produce energy via aerobic metabolism. These mechanisms all work together to encourage weight gain and return to your original weight. To be a successful weight loser and maintain your new weight, minimize the magnitude of these compensatory adaptations by losing weight relatively slowly, using small energy deficits. In other words, don't drastically change your life all at once by eating much less than what you're used to and running much more than what you're used to in an attempt to lose 5 or more pounds per week. It's hard to sustain that drastic lifestyle. Let the drastic changes happen over time, a little at a time, so that they become habits and so that your metabolism and central nervous system have time to adjust and adapt to your changing weight. Running as a habit is *very* effective at keeping your weight off once you have lost it, because running steers the calories you consume away from energy storage and into energy use. People who don't exercise are not only more likely to gain weight, it is inevitable that they will.

◆ ◆ ◆ ◆ ◆

LIKE BORN-AGAIN CHRISTIANS finding Christ, successful weight losers often talk about weight loss as if they are reborn. "I can truly say that finding fitness showed me who I really am," says Jessica Skarzynski, who blogs about her weight loss at jessrunshappy.com. "I gained the majority of my weight in college as I was discovering my adult identity, and while I was enjoying my new freedoms and figuring out what I wanted to do with my life, I always felt physically restrained because I was so much bigger than other 21-year-olds.

"Once I started to lose the weight, my self-esteem increased and my mood improved. The only way I can describe it is that I finally felt like I fit my body. And, best of all, my anxiety subsided enough to allow me to go off my medication within that first year.

I learned that with hard work, dedication, and mental grit, I can overcome pretty much anything life can throw my way."

But it hasn't all been easy. One night, after she had already lost a lot of weight, she got together with some of her overweight college friends whom she hadn't seen since before her weight loss. After the gang ordered another round of appetizers, she turned the plate down, saying she didn't want to go overboard. One friend replied sarcastically, "Oh, please, the skinny bitch needs to watch her weight!" Everyone had a good laugh.

"I was shocked," Jessica says. "I know she meant it jokingly, but the way she said it made me feel like she viewed me as a traitor for losing weight. I never expected someone's opinion of me to shift so drastically. To the people who didn't really know me very well, I didn't look like the same girl—so I wasn't treated like her anymore."

At 32, Jessica is 105 pounds lighter than she was when she was 21. After losing 40 pounds in that first year, it took 3 more years to lose another 65. She has maintained that weight loss since 2009, all with running. She's completed countless races, including two sprint triathlons and, with her half marathon a few days after our interview, seven half marathons. "I ran my first race in 2010 and haven't looked back," she says. "I have no intention of stopping."

When I ask Jessica what advice she has for others, she speaks with the eloquence and perspective of someone much wiser than her years. "I know from experience that it's so easy to backslide once you've had a day, week, or month of bad eating and no exercise. But every passing minute is a chance to turn it all around. You have the power to take control one meal, one snack, and one moment at a time. Every time you eat something or have a few minutes of free time, you have a choice to make: Go for easy, unhealthy food and do nothing, or make a healthy choice and move that body.

"I am by no means perfect," Jessica admits. "I'm a firm believer in 'everything in moderation' and never deny myself chocolate or cake or some other yummy treat when my body is really craving it. I used to be the girl who claimed that 'I don't run unless I'm being chased,' and I literally trapped myself in my own body with anxiety and weight gain. But 10 years and 100-plus pounds later, I really am living proof. I spent most of my teen and adult life hiding from what I could become, and once I conquered that fear and did something about it, I finally found the courage I needed to change. I became an athlete, a runner; I became the me I always knew I was!

"I never set out on this journey, saying 'I'm going to lose 100 pounds,'" Jessica says, "so it never seemed difficult to lose weight. My only goal was to be healthier, and that just naturally happened as I continued on my journey. The changes I've gone through by going from a size 22/24 to a size 8/10 in 4 years affected a lot more than my closet, and I'm interested in exploring all of them!"

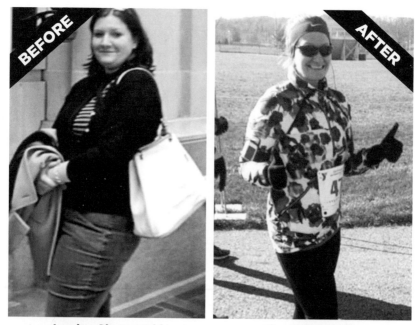

Jessica Skarzynski at 275 pounds.

Skarzynski now, at 170 pounds.

CHAPTER 3

Running Right

"YOU JUST HAVE TO WANT YOUR LIFE TO CHANGE SO BADLY THAT YOU WILL DO ANYTHING TO GET THERE."

F YOU WATCHED SPORTS ON TELEVISION in New Orleans between 2006 and 2011, you probably saw some of Janel Evans's work. A producer for Cox Sports Television, she produced a variety of programming, from local high school football games to the New Orleans Saints' program, *Outside the Huddle*, which highlights the community activities of the Saints organization and its players. It was a demanding job, requiring long hours and a 50-mile commute from her home in Covington, Louisiana. She lived on fast food and didn't exercise. She even had a list of favorite fast-food meals.

In 2011, at age 35, she changed jobs, and shortly after giving birth to her second daughter, suddenly found herself working only minutes from her home with an abundance of free time on her hands. "All of the excuses I had made were suddenly gone," she says, "so I joined a gym to finally take control of my weight." At the gym, she got a physical assessment and found out that she weighed 276 pounds.

◆ ◆ ◆ ◆ ◆

ALTHOUGH THERE ARE SOME DIFFERING THEORIES on running technique, no one really knows if there is a "best" way to run. Any "best" way is likely slightly different for each runner, because every runner subconsciously runs as efficiently as he or she possibly can. Your body is not going to do what is inefficient. Running biomechanics are influenced by skeletal alignment, flexibility, and strength. If you try to change your biomechanics without changing the factors that influence it, you can get injured. If you're a new runner, practicing the skill of running will make running easier, help prevent injuries, and enable you to run longer and faster, all of which will help you lose more weight. To be a better runner and lose weight for the long term, start by running better.

> **" TO BE A BETTER RUNNER AND LOSE WEIGHT FOR THE LONG TERM, START BY RUNNING BETTER."**

BASIC POINTS OF RUNNING TECHNIQUE

Running has an under-recognized neural component, perhaps because it seems like such a simple movement that we all make as toddlers. But to run well, there's actually a lot going on with your central nervous system and your muscles. Just as the repetition of the walking movements decreases the jerkiness of a toddler's walk to the point that it becomes smooth, the repetition of specific running movements ingrains your muscle fiber recruitment patterns and enables a more efficient application of muscular force, making you a smoother runner.

Acknowledging that there is no ideal running technique that

should be adopted by every runner, there are certain things you should strive for when you run to a leaner and fitter you:

◆ Land with your foot and leg as directly underneath your hips as possible. This will enable you to roll from one stride into the next instead of braking your forward motion. With the large amount of cushioning that most running shoes have, it is very common to land on the heel. Landing on the heel when running slowly is okay, but don't overstride by landing sharply with the heel and leg out in front of your body. This will cause you to decelerate and to land on the ground with a lot of force that your joints will have to absorb. The faster you run, the more you'll naturally land toward the forefoot.

◆ Make a conscious effort to run as lightly as possible over the ground, feeling your feet land directly under your body and springing (but not bouncing) off the ground with each step.

What about your arms? Are they important when you run? I'm glad you asked. Of course your arms are important because they balance your legs. As Isaac Newton taught us, for every action there is an equal and opposite reaction. Quick, powerful arm movements mean quick, powerful leg movements. Move your arms the wrong way, and your legs will move the wrong way to compensate. After you have practiced how to move your legs and how to land with your feet directly beneath your hips, you can focus on the motion of your arms.

◆ Hold your arms close to your body and swing them back and forth from your shoulders like a pendulum, with your forearms swinging at a slight angle toward your body.

◆ Keep your elbows bent at 90 degrees or slightly less through the entire movement.

◆ Don't allow your arms to cross over the midline of your chest. When your arms cross your chest, your torso starts twisting, causing undesirable sideways movement.

◆ Keep the palms of your hands facing your body and relax your hands as if you're gently holding a potato chip. But don't break the potato chip! Be gentle. (And don't eat the potato chip because you're trying to run your fat off!) Relax your hands and arms so there is no tension in your upper body.

◆ Swing your arms with quick, compact movements. Your legs do what your arms do, so quick arms mean quick legs.

◆ To run faster, increase the cadence of your arms. Move your arms back and forth faster from your shoulder, but keep the movements controlled and compact.

◆ Don't lean forward from your hips. Keep your torso as quiet as possible. The only things that should be moving are your arms (from the shoulder joint) and your legs.

RUNNING DRILLS

Like any other skill, from playing the piano to riding a bicycle, running expertise comes through constant repetition. Drills that specifically target each part of the running motion improve your running technique and coordination as your central nervous system ingrains the movements. Drills also increase specific flexibility because their dynamic action moves your joints through an exaggerated range of motion.

When doing the running drills in this chapter, take time to recover fully between each set and each drill to avoid fatigue and maintain correct form. It's better to not do the drills at all than to do them with improper form, since that will only create and ingrain bad habits. Be deliberate about all of the movements and focus on what you're doing. These drills and the proper running technique that they aim to produce will help you run effectively, which will make your runs easier. People get turned off from running all too often because they slog through runs that they perceive as difficult. Wouldn't you rather glide through runs that you perceive as easy and enjoyable?

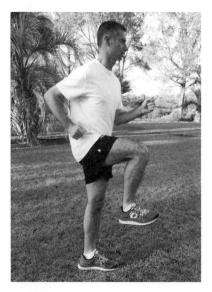

High-Knee Walk

Walk like you are a member of a marching band, raising your knee until your thigh is parallel to the ground, creating a 90-degree angle at your hip. Keep your lower leg perpendicular to your thigh so that your knee is also at 90 degrees, and point your toes up so your ankle is at 90 degrees. Lower your leg so that it comes down directly underneath your hips, landing with your midfoot. Use quick, sharp movements. Do 2 to 4 sets of about 30 to 40 meters.

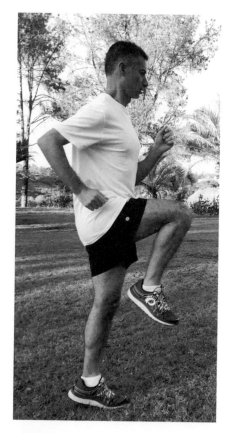

High-Knee Skip

This drill is similar to the high-knee walk but is performed while skipping, raising your knee until your thigh is parallel to the ground, creating a 90-degree angle at your hip. As you raise your knee, hop with the other leg. As with the high-knee walk, keep your lower leg perpendicular to your thigh so that your knee is also at 90 degrees, and point your toes up so your ankle is at 90 degrees. Lower your leg so that it comes down directly underneath your hips, landing with your midfoot. Use quick, sharp movements. Do 2 to 4 sets of about 30 to 40 meters.

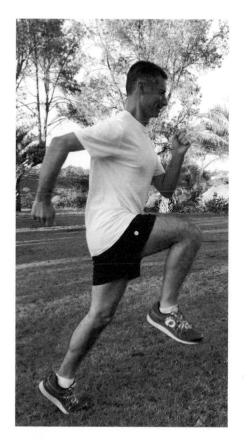

High-Knee Run

This drill is similar to the high-knee walk and skip but is performed while running. Move your legs up and down as fast as you
can, like a sewing machine. Think of the ground as hot coals, picking your leg up as soon as it touches the ground. As with the other
drills, raise your knee until your thigh is parallel to the ground,
creating a 90-degree angle at your hip. Keep your lower leg perpendicular to your thigh so that your knee is also at 90 degrees,
and point your toes up so your ankle is at 90 degrees. Lower your
leg so that it comes down directly underneath your hips. Remain
on the ball of your foot. Run tall and don't lean back. Use quick,
sharp movements. Do 2 to 4 sets of about 30 to 40 meters.

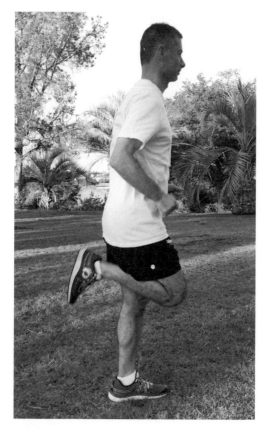

Butt Kickers

Moving your legs fast, keep your knees stationary and flex your leg behind you until the heel of your shoe flicks the back of your butt. Lower your leg so that it comes down directly underneath your hips. Remain on the ball of your foot. Use quick, sharp movements. Do 2 to 4 sets of about 30 to 40 meters.

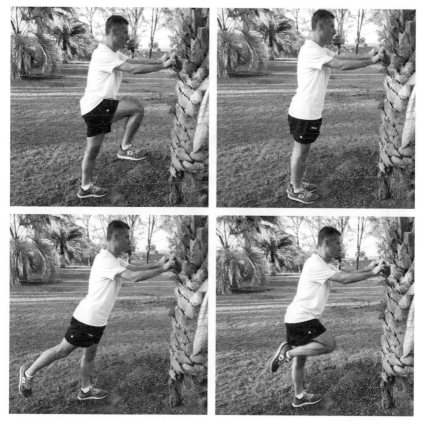

Running Leg Cycle

All of the former drills come into play in this drill, which takes your legs through the entire running motion. Lean slightly against a fence, pole, or tree, but don't bend at the waist. Start with your leg raised and your hip and knee at 90 degrees (like the high-knee walk drill), then lower your leg and sweep it behind you, extending your leg at the hip. Then, bend your knee and pull your knee to the front of your body until your hip is again at 90 degrees in the start position (also with 90-degree angles at your knee and ankle), and repeat the motion. Think, "Land, push off, pull your knee through to the front. Land, push off, pull through." Do 2 to 3 sets of 20 reps with each leg.

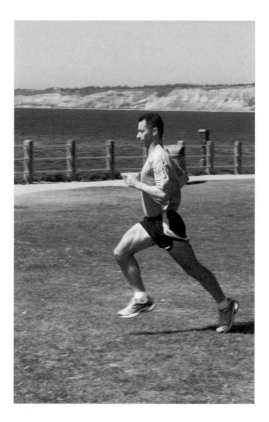

Strides

Strides are short, quick, controlled-effort sprints for about 10 to 20 seconds. They give you a chance to practice the above drills while you run. Aim for a fast, smooth feeling. Don't push yourself to go fast—they shouldn't feel difficult. Rather, relax and focus on moving your legs fast to increase stride rate and extending your legs behind you from your hip to increase stride length. Do a handful of them each time, perhaps 4 to 8. Take as much time as you need between each one to feel recovered. Run strides on flat ground. After practicing the drills on a few occasions, incorporate strides into the routine by immediately following each drill with a couple of strides for about 10 seconds to ingrain the movements of the drills into your running.

RUNNING WORKOUTS

People who don't run often ask me how to start running, as if there is some special wisdom that needs to be learned, like what a Jedi Master learns from Yoda. Those people are always surprised when I say, in my best Yoda voice, "Just start running, you will."

Running, or even the *thought* of running, can be very intimidating to many people. The truth is that running may be the easiest activity to do. You start running by putting on a pair of running shoes, stepping outside your door, and running. It's really that easy. If you're out of shape, don't worry. So what if you can't run for more than 30 seconds? You don't have to run like a Kenyan. Only Kenyans have to run like Kenyans. Run for 30 seconds, if that's all you can do. If you can run longer, run longer. Then walk for 5 minutes. But don't take a sunset stroll on the beach; walk as though you are late to catch your flight. Walk with intention, the intention to burn the fat and become leaner and fitter. After 5 minutes of fast walking, run again for 30 seconds or as long as you can. Keep doing that run-walk-run pattern until 30 minutes have passed. Then do the same thing tomorrow. Over time, as your body adapts and your fitness improves, you can run for 60 seconds at a time. Then 2 minutes. Then 4 minutes. Before you know it, you'll be running your fat off for the entire 30 minutes.

And that's how you start running.

When progressing from walking to running, slowly and consistently increase how much you run and the speed at which you run, but start with increasing how much. You must be patient—there are no shortcuts to becoming a runner and there are no shortcuts to weight loss. Just as with many other big projects in your life, losing weight is a process. It didn't take you 6 months to put on all the extra weight, so don't expect it to take 6 months to remove it. You must work diligently every day at the process. Progress slowly and give your body a chance to adapt. You don't have to rush through life or your weight-loss journey at someone else's pace; you have only to take life at the pace that is right for you.

If you're already a runner, or at least someone who runs, you need to go beyond basic running to lose the fat. You need to ramp up your training. That means running more and running faster. More running and faster running are beautiful things, because they don't just help you lose weight and keep it off; they also make you a more proficient runner.

So what kind of running should you do to lose the most weight in the shortest amount of time? You can run slowly, you can run fast, you can run for a long time, you can run for a short time. Or any combination of these. By running at different paces, from very slow to very fast, you become a more complete runner even if you never run a race. By becoming a complete runner, you can handle more volume and more intensity, and that will go very far to improving your fitness, creating vitality in your life, and guaranteeing that you'll meet your weight-loss goals.

Because running is often measured in distance (miles or kilometers, depending on where in the world you live), it is easy to measure your progress. For example, you may run 5 miles the first week and 20 miles per week 3 months later! If you're a more advanced runner, you may start with 30 miles per week and run 60 miles per week 3 months later! That's major progress and it burns lots of calories. And that's empowering.

Unfortunately, fitness is lost quickly. To see results, you need to run consistently. It will take much longer to see results if you run 3 days this week, 2 days next week, 1 day the week after, 0 days the week after that, 2 days the following week, and so on. A single run is not enough. If you run for 1 hour, you may burn 600 to 800 calories, depending on how many miles you cover. That may seem like a lot for 1 day, but if that run were the only one you did the whole week, it won't have a significant impact on your body weight. Daily running grows your bank account of burned calories, which, over time, becomes a significant contributor to weight loss. If you really want to see results, you must be consistent with your running and accumulate a caloric deficit—day after day, week after week, month after month, year after year.

The main reason people don't lose as much weight as they want to is that they don't maintain a large enough caloric deficit. In their review of the exercise and weight-loss research, scientists at Montclair State University in New Jersey and the Pennington Biomedical Research Center in Baton Rouge, Louisiana, concluded that the small amount of weight loss observed from the majority of exercise intervention studies is primarily due to low doses of prescribed exercise energy expenditures compounded by a concomitant increase in caloric intake. In other words, people don't exercise enough and they eat more to compensate for the calories they expend during exercise.

> **" PEOPLE DON'T EXERCISE ENOUGH AND THEY EAT MORE TO COMPENSATE FOR THE CALORIES THEY EXPEND DURING EXERCISE."**

Aerobic Runs

Aerobic running—running that uses oxygen—is the simplest and perhaps most effective way to enhance your body's ability to burn fat. (Unless you are running very fast, as I'll discuss later, almost all running is aerobic running.) How does it do that? Well, as you might remember from high school, inside your muscles are what my biology teacher called "mighty mitochondria." Inside your mitochondria, a complex series of chemical reactions generates energy by oxidizing carbohydrate and fat. This is called the Krebs cycle, named after its discoverer, biochemist and Nobel Prize winner Hans Krebs.

Aerobic running is a potent stimulus to proliferate mitochondria—your cells' oxygen-using factories—which are responsible for everything inside of you that is aerobic—and that's pretty much everything. Initially, when you're out of shape and start to run, you're inefficient and will use a lot of carbohydrate for energy. But through weeks and months of running, you will build up the metabolic machinery—the mitochondria and Krebs cycle—needed to burn fat instead of carbohydrate. This is one of the hallmark adaptations of aerobic exercise. A low supply of carbohydrate is threatening to your muscles' survival because carbohydrate is their preferred fuel, so your body adapts to running by relying more on fat, thereby delaying the use of carbohydrate and assuaging the threat. Ingenious!

The connection between mitochondria and a muscle's capacity to consume oxygen, first made by Dr. John Holloszy in 1967 in the muscles of treadmill-running laboratory rats at the Washington University School of Medicine, has provided much insight into the adaptability of skeletal muscle. Generally, the greater the demand, the greater the adaptations—run more miles, make more mitochondria. More mitochondria means a greater capacity to use oxygen. A greater capacity to use oxygen means you burn more calories. (Remember from the calculation in Chapter 1 that for every liter of oxygen you consume, you burn 5 calories.)

Running more aerobic miles each week is the most straightforward way to burn more calories, although it is also the most time consuming. It may not feel so easy to run more miles if you're currently out of shape, but you'll get there. You burn about 110 calories per mile, give or take, depending on your body weight and the amount of oxygen you consume when you run, so if you run 5 to 10 more miles per week, you'll burn about an extra 550 to 1,100 calories per week.

Although many different types of aerobic exercise can help you lose weight, running, because of its huge calorie burn, is better at reducing body weight and body mass index in men and women compared to equivalent amounts of any other type of exercise. The reduced body fat you'll get from running also enables you to exercise more and at a higher intensity, which burns even more calories.

Long Runs

Long runs are great for burning calories, and for discovering the meaning of life. There aren't many problems that can't be solved by running 20 miles. Of course, you don't have to run that far unless you're training for a marathon (or want to discover the meaning of life), but running longer than you usually do will burn more calories than you usually do. It will also make your muscles more fuel efficient, training them to rely more on fat. Do one long run per week that is significantly longer than any of your other runs. Run slowly enough that you can complete the distance. If you have to stop and walk, then stop and walk. The point is to run (or run/walk) longer than what you're used to; if you go too fast in the beginning and have to stop the run, that will defeat the purpose.

A 10-mile run burns about 1,100 calories, regardless of how fast or slowly you run. Pace only matters if you run for time rather than distance. For example, if you have 30 minutes to run, the faster you run for those 30 minutes, the more calories you'll burn because you will cover more distance in those 30 minutes. If you run 3 miles, you'll burn the same number of calories whether you run the 3 miles in 15 minutes or in 30 minutes. The more you weigh, the more calories you'll burn each mile you run, because it costs more oxygen to transport a heavier person.

The longer you run, or even walk, the more and longer your

metabolic rate is elevated afterward. One study published in *Medicine & Science in Sports & Exercise* found that walking for 60 minutes at a brisk pace resulted in a higher postworkout metabolic rate than did walking at the same pace for 20 or 40 minutes. Also, the longer people walked, the longer it took for their metabolic rate to return to pre-exercise levels, taking 2, 3.5, and 7.5 hours following the 20-, 40-, and 60-minute walks. In another study published in the *Canadian Journal of Sport Sciences*, postworkout metabolic rate more than doubled when the amount of time people exercised increased from 30 to 45 minutes and increased more than fivefold after exercising for 60 minutes. Long runs burn more calories both during and after the runs.

Tempo Runs

Tempo runs are comfortably hard runs at the upper end of being purely aerobic. The pace corresponds to a physiological marker called the *lactate threshold,* which represents the fastest pace that you can sustain aerobically without a significant anaerobic (oxygen-independent) contribution. You can think of tempo runs as hard but controlled aerobic running. On these runs, don't try to push the pace. Rather, run at your correct tempo pace, keep it aerobic, and work on holding that pace for longer periods of time. (You'll learn how to figure out your tempo pace in Chapter 4.) Tempo runs, because of their faster pace, burn more calories in the same time as the more comfortable aerobic runs.

Aerobic Power Runs

Aerobic power runs are fast-paced runs that correspond to the maximum rate at which your muscles can consume oxygen. To understand what aerobic power means, let's go for a run. Don't worry—we'll start slowly. Your breathing is comfortable and shallow. Heart rate is elevated but not noticeable. You can have a conversation with me. You're running at a pace at which you can run forever. Now let's pick up the pace. You start to breathe more heavily. You have to stop talking after a couple of sentences to breathe. Your heart rate rises. Blood flow to your muscles increases. Your muscles consume more oxygen. Now pick up the pace some more. The volume of oxygen you consume continues to increase to keep up with the demand of the run. Keep running faster until you're revving your aerobic engine as fast as it can go and you're huffing and puffing. Our conversation stops. Your muscles are consuming as much oxygen as they can. This pace corresponds to the popular physiological marker VO_2max, which literally means the maximum volume of oxygen your body consumes per minute.

When you run at your VO_2max, your cardiovascular system is working as hard as it can—your heart rate, stroke volume (the volume of blood your heart pumps with each beat), and cardiac output (the volume of blood your heart pumps each minute) all reach their maximum values. Many people who don't exercise are afraid of getting their heart rate too high because they think that it is dangerous for their hearts when in fact it is one of the best ways to strengthen their hearts. Your VO_2max represents the size of your aerobic engine and is considered the single best indicator of your aerobic fitness. The bigger your engine, the more and faster oxygen can be consumed, and the greater your aerobic power.

Because VO_2max occurs at a faster speed than your lactate threshold (the pace of your tempo runs), aerobic power runs are actually somewhat anaerobic (oxygen-independent). By contrast, the lactate threshold is still purely aerobic and represents the fraction of your VO_2max that you can sustain. When you run *faster* than the pace at which you reach your VO_2max, much of the energy supporting that pace is produced by anaerobic (oxygen-independent) means.

Aerobic power runs focus on giving you a bigger aerobic engine. They are like strength training for your heart. When you improve the capacity of your cardiovascular system—your heart's ability to pump blood and oxygen to the active muscles and to your other organs—you improve VO_2max. One of the best methods to increase VO_2max is with interval training, during which you run hard and fast at the pace that corresponds to your maximum heart rate for 3 to 5 minutes and then "recover" by running at a slower pace for 3 to 5 minutes. This type of workout, which is demanding, is one of the best workouts you can do to improve your cardiovascular conditioning and burn a lot of calories.

Anaerobic Runs

Let's face it, when you first start a running program, any running pace is hard. You're huffing and puffing and nearly blowing your house down. When you get fit, however, you increase the range of speeds at which you can run. You'll have slow paces, moderate paces, fast paces, and paces so tough you'll feel like you're tethered to a Kenyan.

Contrary to slow aerobic running, fast anaerobic running does not use oxygen. When you run fast for short periods, like the kind of sprinting you did as a kid on the playground at recess, the activity becomes anaerobic, or oxygen-independent, because your cardiovascular system becomes unable to supply oxygen quickly enough to meet the metabolic demands of your muscles. In other words, the demand for oxygen at the pace you're running is greater than its supply. Lots of side effects occur when this happens, all of which cause you to fatigue rapidly and slow down.

Most people, especially when they start a running program, are afraid to run fast. They think they're going to blow up or something. But running fast comes with its own set of internal changes. When you rev your metabolic engine as fast as it will go, it increases the number of enzymes that catalyze the chemical reactions in your non-oxygen-using metabolic pathways. One of those pathways is called *glycolysis,* literally the breaking down of glucose. Anaerobic running relies exclusively on glucose for energy, which teaches your body to become better at using glucose rather than storing it as fat. If you rev your metabolic engine on a regular basis such that you make your muscles rely on glucose, the carbohydrate calories you eat won't get stored as fat because they will be used to replace the glucose you have used when running.

Running fast also does a lot for your muscles. It recruits your powerful fast-twitch muscle fibers, which enhances your strength and makes your muscles look better on your body. Track sprinters have some of the nicest bodies around.

Interval Runs

Once the training secret of the world's best runners, interval training has become the new buzz term in the fitness industry. It seems as if everyone is doing it, from competitive athletes to grandma next door. In an interval workout, you alternate periods of faster running to get your heart pumping with periods of slower jogging (or walking) to recover. Interval workouts are a fast and potent way to get fit and lose weight because you can exercise at a higher intensity when you intersperse the exercise with periods of recovery.

While many athletes used interval training in the first half of the twentieth century, it was distance runner Emil Zatopek of the former Czechoslovakia, winner of the 10K at the 1948 Olympics and the 5K, 10K, and marathon at the 1952 Olympics, who popularized this method of training. However, it wasn't until the 1960s that famous Swedish physiologist Per-Olaf Åstrand discovered, using a stationary bicycle in a laboratory, what many coaches and runners already knew—that by breaking up a set amount of work into smaller segments, you can perform the work at a higher intensity. For example, you can run five 4-minute segments with breaks faster than you can run 20 minutes continuously; you can run ten 2-minute segments with breaks faster than you can run five 4-minute segments; and you can run twenty 1-minute segments with breaks faster than you can run ten 2-minute segments. The shorter the time (or distance) you run, the faster you can run the total time (or distance) of the workout. Sounds obvious, but Åstrand's simple observation is the basis for interval training.

Preceding Åstrand's work by 30 years, German coach Waldemar Gerschler and physiologist Hans Reindell of Germany's Freiburg University studied the cardiovascular effects of interval training. As they proved, the stimulus for cardiovascular improvement occurs during the recovery intervals between runs, when the heart rate decreases from an elevated value. Thus, the emphasis of the workout was placed on the recovery interval, prompting Gerschler and Reindell to call it an "interval workout" or "interval training." Gerschler and Reindell's original interval training method consisted of running periods from 30 to 70 seconds at an intensity that elevated the heart rate to 170 to 180 beats per minute, followed by recovery periods to allow the heart rate to drop to 120 beats per minute, signifying the readiness to perform the next running period.

During the recovery interval, the heart rate declines quickly because the runner has stopped running fast, but there is a lot of blood returning to the heart and lungs to get rid of the carbon dioxide and pick up more oxygen. Since the heart rate declines rapidly (and declines faster the more fit you are because fit people's hearts are better at pumping blood), there's more time for blood to fill the left ventricle of the heart to accommodate the large volume of blood returning to the heart, which causes a brief increase in stroke volume (the volume of blood your heart pumps with each beat). Since stroke volume peaks during the recovery interval, the more recovery intervals you have during a workout, the more opportunity for your heart's maximum stroke volume and the capacity of your cardiovascular system to improve. Interval workouts improve your cardiovascular fitness quickly, which is great news for busy people who don't want to spend 2 hours in the gym. Interval workouts manipulate four variables:

1. Time (or distance) of each running period
2. Pace of each running period
3. Time of each recovery interval
4. Number of repetitions

With so many possible combinations of these four variables, you have nearly unlimited potential to vary your workouts and never get bored. Although runners tend to pay more attention to the pace and distance of each running period, the benefit from interval workouts occurs from a combination of running and recovery. The recovery intervals are very important to the design and effectiveness of the workouts. That combination of running and recovery is what makes interval runs different from continuous runs.

The *Run Your Fat Off* running menus include a variety of interval runs, including hill runs, aerobic power runs, and anaerobic runs.

Hill Runs

Many runners have a love-hate relationship with hills. Hills are tough, but the payoff is extraordinary. The feel of your heart pounding in your chest and your shortness of breath at the top of a hill attest to what hills can do for your cardiovascular system. It's relatively easy to drive up your heart rate when you run hills. Hills also give your legs and butt a great workout as your muscles work harder to run against gravity. Because you use so much muscle when running hills, you burn a lot of calories. You'll see in the running menus in Chapter 4 that you can do several different kinds of hill runs to keep things interesting: runs during which the incline keeps getting steeper; runs during which the incline gets steeper and then declines; and runs during which the incline keeps changing.

Double Runs

An advanced weight-loss strategy, running twice per day allows you to increase your daily and weekly mileage over what you

TREADMILL RUNS

I once coached a woman who started running in her late twenties. She told me that when she first started running, she was intimidated about running outside, so she started on the treadmill instead.

The original modern version of the treadmill was first used for exercise in 1952, when Robert Bruce and Wayne Quinton at the University of Washington in Seattle had their patients walk on it so they could monitor their heart function. It has since become the most popular piece of cardio equipment in the gym. Many beginner runners start running on a treadmill because there's a certain comfort about the controlled environment of the treadmill. It's safe. If anything happens, you're not miles from home. You can't get lost on a treadmill other than in your thoughts.

Treadmill running may also feel easier than running outdoors because you use less energy and burn fewer normally run, which increases the number of calories you'll burn. Although it takes more time out of your day to run twice, it's easier, both physically and psychologically, to run 2 miles in the morning and 4 miles in the evening (for a total of 6 miles) than it is to run 6 miles (or even 5 miles) all at once.

Research shows that double workouts are not just effective for burning calories during the workouts; they are also good for burning calories afterward. Splitting your daily run into two shorter runs results in two separate elevations in your post-workout metabolic rate, which gives you two opportunities to burn more calories during the day. One study had women run

calories when compared to running over ground, particularly at faster speeds. When you run on a treadmill, there is no air resistance and your muscles don't have to work as hard because the treadmill belt pulls your leg back as it lands. Treadmills are also a great way to do specific workouts, like hill runs and tempo runs, because of the ability to manually manipulate the grade and speed.

You may feel self-conscious going to the gym to run on a treadmill, though, especially if you're overweight. But don't be intimidated by the fit people you see there who wear spandex and love to show off their perfect bodies. Don't worry about other people staring at you. Chances are, those people started off as overweight and out of shape, too, and they're now too involved with their own workouts to pay attention to you.

for 50 minutes one day and twice for 25 minutes at the same intensity another day. Even though the total amount of time spent running was the same, the increase in postworkout metabolic rate was higher after the two workouts when compared to the increase after the single workout. By running twice per day, you get two metabolic bangs for your buck.

Of course, I'm not saying you should run twice per day every day; few people have time for that. But it's worth trying a couple of times each week if you can. If you don't want to run twice per day, try doing some other exercise. For example, run 2 or 3 miles in the morning and do either another cardio workout or resistance workout in the evening. No matter what type of exercise you do, the more you exercise, the more calories you'll burn. Plus, by having two acute increases in your postworkout metabolic rate, you'll burn even more.

Supplemental Workouts

Supplemental workouts include nonrunning activities, like cross-training, resistance training, and stretching. While these activities may not have a direct impact on your running, they can improve your overall fitness and burn calories on days you don't run, increase muscular strength and flexibility, and reduce the chance of injury. You can think of supplemental workouts as exercises and activities that prepare you for more formal running workouts and enable you to handle greater amounts of running.

Cross-Training

If you're a beginner runner, you won't be able to run every day at first. But since you have to eat every day, you need to fill in the gaps between runs with other exercise to keep the weight coming off.

Cross-training, like swimming, cycling, and circuit training, is any cardiovascular activity or exercise that supplements your running. Although cross-training won't directly make you a better runner or burn as many calories, it has certain benefits:

◆ **It increases aerobic fitness apart from running.** If you're a beginner runner, you can't expect to run 30 or 40 miles or more per week. Getting your running volume that high takes time. So, on the days you don't run, you can supplement your running with cross-training to boost your aerobic fitness without the physical stress (and injury risk) of running more.

◆ **It helps you lose weight.** In addition to increasing aerobic fitness, cross-training will add to your weekly calorie burn, which can contribute to your weight-loss goals, and losing weight makes running easier.

◆ **It maintains cardiovascular fitness while injured.** An injury often prevents you from running, but cross-training with a different activity that doesn't directly put stress on the injured body part enables you to stay fit while your injury heals so that you're not completely out of shape when you start running again.

◆ **It works different muscles.** Cross-training helps strengthen nonrunning muscles and gives your running muscles some recovery. Focus your cross-training on your nonrunning muscles, such as the muscles of your upper body.

◆ **It reduces the risk of overuse injuries.** Cross-training varies the intensity and volume of your workouts and spreads the stress across different muscles.

◆ **It boosts recovery after tough workouts.** Cross-training the day after an interval workout or long run brings blood full of oxygen and nutrients to your muscles without the extra stress to your running muscles and joints.

◆ **It increases flexibility.** Running a lot can decrease range of motion, causing certain muscles, like hamstrings and calves, to tighten. Cross-training with activities different from running can increase flexibility by moving your limbs through larger ranges of motion.

If you are very overweight and have orthopedic issues that may initially limit your running, cross-training is a great way to jump-start your exercise program and start burning calories. Many people have to lose some weight before they begin running. That's okay. You're in this for the long haul anyway. Running will be there for you when you are ready.

Resistance Training

When I was in eighth grade, I broke the school record for chin-ups. I still have the certificate of achievement from the school's principal proudly displayed on my wall. I still brag about the accomplishment to others. It doesn't matter that it was so many years ago or that some tough kid has probably come along since to break my record. At the time, I had the strongest biceps and forearms in junior high. I used chin-ups to show off to the girls in class. My mother even bought a chin-up bar and attached it to my bedroom door frame so I could train at home. I did chin-ups every day. What I learned from doing chin-ups (besides that I could get attention from girls) is that there's power in strength.

Over the years, I've gotten away from resistance training (also often called strength or weight training) in favor of more running.

I have a friend who thinks I have some philosophical aversion to resistance training. As a hard-core weight lifter and successful group fitness instructor who has created many workout DVDs, she tells me that I'm unbalanced because all I do is run. Although I do choose to run as my daily workout, I keep promising her that I will one day incorporate some upper-body resistance training to make my biceps as big as my calves. The truth is that I have no aversion, philosophical or otherwise, to resistance training. It just doesn't provide me with the same satisfaction as running. When you get hooked on running, you'll likely feel the same way.

But my friend has a good point. You don't want a house built on shaky ground. If your foundation is weak from years of inactivity, there's less chance that your muscles, bones, and tendons will be able to withstand the stress of running. Because muscles stabilize joints, joint injuries can occur if the muscles surrounding them are weak. Before you start a running program, you may want to do some resistance training to improve the strength of your feet and ankles, hip abductors and adductors, quadriceps, calves, and trunk. This will help support your joints and reduce your chance of getting injured. Let's face it: If you get injured, you'll be sitting on your couch reading *Runner's World* magazine instead of running yourself.

When you lose weight through diet alone, you lose fat (which is great) and muscle (which is not great). Exercise maintains muscle mass so that most of the weight you lose is fat (which is really great). Although running is one of the best exercises to lose fat, resistance training does a better job at maintaining muscle mass. If you include some resistance training into your running program, you can prevent a loss of muscle mass as you lose weight.

Resistance training can also help you lose fat, in part due to the extra calories you'll burn. For example, in a study at Penn State University, 35 overweight men were randomly assigned to one of four groups: (1) diet only, (2) diet plus aerobic exercise, (3) diet plus aerobic exercise plus resistance training, or (4) control group. The individuals in the diet plus aerobic exercise group used a variety of exercise machines, including treadmill, stationary bike, rower, and stair climber, for 30 to 50 minutes at 70 to 80 percent of their maximum heart rate. Those in the diet plus aerobic exercise plus resistance training group also included a variety of resistance exercises consisting of one to three sets of moderate to heavy weights. Both exercise groups followed their specific exercise intervention three times per week for 12 weeks. The individuals in the control group did nothing.

After 12 weeks, all three diet intervention groups showed significant and similar reductions in body weight: 21.21, 19.78, and 21.78 pounds, respectively. However, while 69 percent of the weight lost in the diet-only group was fat, the diet plus aerobic exercise group lost 78 percent of its weight as fat while the diet plus aerobic exercise plus resistance training group lost 97 percent of its weight as fat. That's huge!

In addition to building your foundation and maintaining muscle, resistance training has many other benefits:

◆ **Improved physical appearance and self-image:** Like an artist molding a piece of clay, resistance training, within genetic limitations, can sculpt the way you look, making you feel more confident.

◆ **Greater endurance:** Increasing your muscle strength reduces the percentage of your maximal strength required for each muscle contraction when you run, which delays fatigue and increases your endurance.

◆ **Increased muscle power:** Because your feet are in contact with the ground for only a fraction of a second with each step, your muscles don't have enough time to generate maximal force; producing as much force as you can against the ground as quickly as possible is far more important. By increasing your muscle power, your muscles become better at producing force quickly, so you have stronger muscle contractions in a shorter amount of time.

◆ **Improved communication between your brain and your muscles:** Resistance training does just as much for your brain as it does for your muscles. Lifting weights trains your central nervous system to recruit your muscle fibers quicker. It's like changing from a dial-up modem to broadband for your Internet connection. The faster your brain recruits your muscle fibers, the faster your muscles work and the better you'll run.

◆ **Improved posture and coordination:** Stronger muscles help you move better and maintain correct running posture when you fatigue, which helps you run better. Apart from running, it also improves your physical frame, which is what you present to the world every time you walk into a room.

◆ **Increase in muscle tissue and prevention of loss of muscle tissue that accompanies aging:** One of the defining changes to your body as you age is a loss of muscle mass, which reduces your muscle strength and power. Resistance training can prevent that loss of muscle mass and even replace muscle you've already lost so you can regain your strength and power.

◆ **Increased bone density:** Bones become weaker as you age, increasing your risk of osteoporosis, a common degenerative bone condition. Resistance training has a potent effect on bones, making them denser, which reduces your risk of running-related bone injuries like stress fractures.

Although it's not hard to convince a man to lift weights—most men wish they could have a chest like a caveman, symbolic of their strength—women are often more reluctant to do so because they often think that weight lifting will make them look too bulky or too masculine. Whether or not you get bigger muscles, called *hypertrophy,* depends on three factors—gender, genetics, and training intensity. Males acquire larger muscles than do females due to a greater amount of testosterone, which influences the ability to build new protein in muscles. Genetically, some people have more testosterone and more of the powerful and strong fast-twitch muscle fibers than do others, which enables them to get bigger muscles more easily. Fast-twitch muscle fibers (which you use for strong, powerful anaerobic and sprinting activities) have more mass and can produce more force than slow-twitch muscle fibers (which you use for aerobic and endurance activities) and can hypertrophy more easily. For a woman to get big muscles, she would have to have an unusually high amount of testosterone and many fast-twitch muscle fibers, the fibers most suited for muscle growth and strength. That leaves training intensity as the only one of the three factors that you can control. When you lift heavy weights and do other anaerobic running like sprinting, there is some muscle breakdown, which leads to muscle growth. But that muscle growth won't make a woman look like a man; it will make her look more defined. And that's sexy.

There is a limit, though, to how much muscle you want to build. Although there is a positive relationship between the amount of muscle you have and your ability to burn calories, adding too much muscle impedes your ability to run because it is difficult to transport. Runners are not muscle bound like bodybuilders. Great runners don't have much muscle mass, yet they can accomplish a huge amount of calorie-burning work. Focus on running to lose weight, but use resistance training as a complement to your running.

If you've never lifted weights before, it can be daunting. When you consider the many different types of exercises, the amount of weight to lift, the number of repetitions and sets, and the amount of rest between sets, you might feel like you need a PhD to understand it all. But really, lifting weights in a gym isn't much different from lifting your 4-year-old to reach the monkey bars; it's just a more formal way to reach your specific weight-loss goals.

The resistance you use to train your muscles can actually come in many forms, including dumbbells, weight machines, medicine balls, resistance bands, even your own body weight. It doesn't really matter which type of resistance you use; your muscles don't know the difference. All they know how to do is to contract to overcome the resistance. To maintain muscle mass as you lose weight and especially to increase it to the extent that you'll have any real impact on your metabolism, your muscles need a stimulus strong enough to cause a lot of protein degradation so that there is a lot of protein synthesis in response. That means putting the pink 1-pound dumbbells away and lifting weights heavy enough to fatigue your muscles. If you are using challenging enough weights, just one or two exercises for each major muscle group is all you need. Given the stress of heavy resistance training, I recommend first spending a few weeks preparing your muscles by using lighter weights, or by circuit training, during which you do a series of resistance exercises, moving from one exercise to the next with little to no rest in between.

◆ ◆ ◆ ◆ ◆

WITH HER NEW GYM MEMBERSHIP, Janel Evans started going to the gym five to six times per week, walking on the treadmill and attending fitness boot camp classes. She also signed up to walk/jog every local 5K she could find—often finishing dead last. "I had two young children when I first started working out, so it was hard to get workouts in, even if I brought them with me," she remembers. "It was also hard to get moving at 276 pounds, but as I saw the weight come off, it was very encouraging."

She also changed her diet. She cut out all fried foods ("next to impossible in New Orleans," she says), processed sugar, and carbonated drinks. One afternoon, as she was walking on the treadmill at the gym, she noticed a woman jump on the treadmill next to her. "I saw her put her drink in the cup holder in front of her. I nearly fell off my treadmill when I saw what her drink was—a java chip frappucino. At 600 calories and 22 grams of fat, I hope she's still on that treadmill! I think people are ignorant about their choices. They just have no idea how bad it is for them," she says.

Six months later, her weight down to 200 pounds, she thought she'd give running a try. After she had lost 100 pounds, someone who had not seen her in months accused her of having gastric bypass surgery. "I wanted to punch her in the face," she says. "If she only knew how many French fries I've passed up, how I didn't have a piece of my own kid's birthday cake, how many times I've replaced my contact lenses because my sweat had ruined them, how many times I've climbed up to the fifth floor of my office building at work to use the restroom even though I work on the second floor, how many times I've gotten out of bed at 5:00 a.m. on a Saturday for a race . . . the list goes on and on. I've earned every ounce of happiness."

In October 2011, she ran her first half marathon at 160 pounds, 116 pounds lighter than she had been 10 months earlier. "If you would have told me on January 1, 2011, that in 10 months I would complete over 30 5Ks, ride in 30-mile bike tours, and run a half marathon, I would have never believed it," she says. A year later, she ran even longer to complete her first marathon. In 2016, she ran another marathon, but this time she ran it after swimming 2.4 miles in the ocean and biking 112 miles—her first Ironman triathlon.

"I think people set out by saying, 'I have 50 or 100 pounds to lose,'" Janel says, "and that is just a big number. When the weight doesn't come off overnight, people get frustrated. I personally set small goals. I would say, 'Okay, when I am 10 pounds down, I will

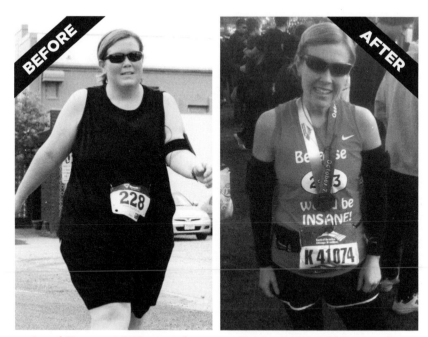

Janel Evans at 276 pounds, walked/jogged 5Ks and came in almost dead last.

Evans now, at 136 pounds, completed an Ironman triathlon.

buy a new pair of shoes. When I am 20 pounds down, I will get a new purse. I was encouraged by meeting small goals and then made bigger goals like signing up for a half marathon, and then a full marathon, and then a sprint triathlon, and then an Ironman."

All told, Janel lost 140 pounds, which took just over a year. She blogs about her running and weight loss at jcrunsnola.blogspot.com. "People ask my weight loss 'secret' all the time. There really wasn't one. You just have to want your life to change so badly that you will do anything to get there. You have to pass on amazing desserts. You have to run when you don't want to. You have to make sacrifices. There's no magic pill. It's purely hard work."

CHAPTER 4

The *Run Your Fat Off* Running Menus

"IT WAS AN OPPORTUNITY TO LEARN NUTRITION, BIOCHEMISTRY, EVEN POLITICS—HOW BIG COMPANIES PREFER TO PROFIT AT THE COST OF OUR HEALTH."

SAN DIEGO, CALIFORNIA, is known for a lot of the "finer" things in life: sunshine, palm trees, postcard views, private yachts, attractive people, millionaires. It's no wonder the city's nickname is America's Finest City. If you hang out at San Diego's Mission Bay on a Sunday morning, you might notice a 6-foot-tall man with short, light brown hair and broad shoulders in a Triathlon Club of San Diego jersey running along the cement boardwalk.

A former software engineer, Roger Leszczynski grew up in New Britain, Connecticut. He runs 10 to 20 miles every morning, bikes 20 to 40 miles during the day, and swims about 1 kilometer every day.

At age 23, he wasn't running, biking, or swimming at all. He weighed 260 pounds. A power weight lifter, his diet consisted of four double cheeseburgers for lunch and pizzas with lots of trans fat. Yes, that's pizzas with an *s*. "I was eating whatever to get big—to lift big weights," he says. "But when I saw someone half my size lifting the same weight as I was lifting, that made me realize that what I thought I was doing right was completely wrong." Then his dad suffered his third heart attack, which made him question his eating habits even more.

"I had high blood pressure and a similar cholesterol level as my dad," he says. "That made me realize that I could be next in line for a heart attack. I cleaned up my diet, removing all of the processed foods and excess carbs, and added cardio to my weight lifting routine. A 10-minute mile was holy hell." Eventually, over time and patience, Roger lost weight, getting faster and stronger. One day at the YMCA, he saw a flyer for a local 5K.

◆ ◆ ◆ ◆ ◆

ENOUGH READING.... It's time to run! In this chapter, you'll find the beginner, intermediate, and advanced running "menus" that make up the *Run Your Fat Off* program, along with "recipes" for each type of run. I designed these menus to maximize your calorie burn and progress from each course of running to the next to help you lose weight and keep it off. There are more than 20 years of running science and experience in each menu, which has worked with hundreds of runners of different levels I have coached. I have included variety in the workouts so you don't get bored.

Choose the menu that's most appropriate for you. If any of the weeks of the menu is especially challenging or you feel like the amount of running is too much, feel free to slow down the progression and repeat a week from the menu before moving on to the next week. Nothing is set in stone here; the important thing is to choose a realistic starting point and progress so you can handle running more volume and more intense workouts. Be consistent with your running—week to week, month to month, year to year. If something comes up that prevents you from doing the prescribed workout, don't worry about it; your weight-loss goal is not determined by a single day of running. It's the accumulation of runs over time that matters. So go ahead and move things around so you can get in as many of the runs as you can each week.

The *Run Your Fat Off* program is not meant to be a short-term fix. It is a lifestyle. There are six courses of training menus laid out in this chapter. Each course can be as many weeks as you need to progress at the rate that is right for you. So repeat a week of each course as many times as you need until it feels comfortable and manageable. After you have completed each course, take a recovery week by decreasing your weekly running volume by about a third before moving on to the next course. After you've enjoyed all six courses, keep running, and keep progressing with the same pattern of volume and intensity outlined in the menus so that you achieve higher levels of fitness and lose more weight. If you're a beginner, complete the beginner menu and then progress to the intermediate menu. If you're already running 3 or 4 hours per week and the beginner menu seems easy to you, start with the intermediate menu and then progress to the advanced menu. As you progress, focus on the process rather than the outcome.

To offer flexibility, you can move runs around each week, as long as you stay consistent and do not miss workouts. For example, if you can't fit in a longer run on Sunday, you can do it on Saturday as long as Friday is not a harder workout day. If Friday is a harder workout, move Friday's workout earlier in the week so you can do the longer run on Saturday. Always have at least one easier day of running after each harder day.

RUN YOUR FAT OFF
BEGINNER MENU

This beginner menu starts in the first course with 3 days of alternating walking and running (5 min walk/5 min run) per week, increasing gradually to 4 days of walk/run (1 min walk/9 min run) per week in Course 6.

After building endurance over the first 4 courses, Course 5 introduces some faster-paced running. Do all of your walk/runs at a brisk walking pace and comfortable running pace for the amount of time listed. Don't worry about being slow. Initially, the important thing is to spend time on your feet, slowly turning yourself into a runner.

As you adapt to running, you'll find that you can run longer before taking a walking break.

Starting with Course 2, Saturday's menu includes two options: off or cross-training.

All Hill Runs and Tempo Runs are served with a 5-minute warm-up walk/run and 5-minute cool-down walk/run.

Course 1

◆ ◆ ◆

MONDAY
Off

TUESDAY
AEROBIC WALK/RUN
30 min: walk 5 min/run 5 min

WEDNESDAY
Off

THURSDAY
AEROBIC WALK/RUN
30 min: walk 5 min/run 5 min

FRIDAY
Off

SATURDAY
Off

SUNDAY
LONG WALK/RUN
40 min: walk 5 min/run 5 min

TOTAL WALK/RUN TIME = 1 HOUR, 40 MINUTES

Recovery Week: For each day above, decrease the amount you walk/run by one-third so that the total walk/run time is 1 hour, 6 minutes.

Course 2

◆ ◆ ◆

MONDAY
Off

TUESDAY
AEROBIC WALK/RUN
20 min: walk 4 min/run 6 min

WEDNESDAY
HILL PYRAMID RUN
5-min warm-up **+**

1 min run at 2%, 4%, 6%, 8%, 6%, 4%, 2% grade
with 1 min walk recovery between runs at 0% grade

+ 5-min cool-down

THURSDAY
Off

FRIDAY
AEROBIC WALK/RUN
40 min: walk 4 min/run 6 min

SATURDAY
Off

or

30-min cross-train

SUNDAY
LONG WALK/RUN
50 min: walk 4 min/run 6 min

TOTAL WALK/RUN TIME = 2 HOURS, 14 MINUTES

Recovery Week: For each day above, decrease the amount you walk/run by one-third so that the total walk/run time is 1 hour, 29 minutes.

Course 3

◆ ◆ ◆

MONDAY
Off

TUESDAY
AEROBIC WALK/RUN
20 min: walk 3 min/run 7 min

WEDNESDAY
HILL LADDER RUN
5-min warm-up **+**

1-min run at 2%, 4%, 6%, 8%, 10%, 12%, 14% grade
with 1-min walk recovery between runs at 0% grade

+ 5-min cool-down

THURSDAY
Off

FRIDAY
AEROBIC WALK/RUN
40 min: walk 3 min/run 7 min

SATURDAY
Off
or
35-min cross-train

SUNDAY
LONG WALK/RUN
60 min: walk 3 min/run 7 min

TOTAL WALK/RUN TIME = 2 HOURS, 24 MINUTES

Recovery Week: For each day above, decrease the amount you walk/run
by one-third so that the total walk/run time is 1 hour, 36 minutes.

Course 4

◆ ◆ ◆

MONDAY
Off

TUESDAY
AEROBIC WALK/RUN
30 min: walk 3 min/run 7 min

WEDNESDAY
HILL MIX RUN
5-min warm-up **+**

1-min run at 4%, 8%, 2%, 6%, 3%, 12%, 9% grade
with 1-min walk recovery between runs at 0% grade

+ 5-min cool-down

THURSDAY
Off

FRIDAY
AEROBIC WALK/RUN
50 min: walk 3 min/run 7 min

SATURDAY
Off
or
40-min cross-train

SUNDAY
LONG WALK/RUN
70 min: walk 3 min/run 7 min

TOTAL WALK/RUN TIME = 2 HOURS, 54 MINUTES

Recovery Week: For each day above, decrease the amount you walk/run by one-third so that the total walk/run time is 1 hour, 56 minutes.

Course 5

♦ ♦ ♦

MONDAY
Off

TUESDAY
AEROBIC WALK/RUN
30 min: walk 2 min/run 8 min

WEDNESDAY
TEMPO RUN
5-min warm-up **+**

4 x 3 min @ tempo pace
with 1-min walk recovery between reps

+ 5-min cool-down

THURSDAY
Off

FRIDAY
AEROBIC WALK/RUN
50 min: walk 2 min/run 8 min + 3 x 10-sec strides

SATURDAY
Off
or
45-min cross-train

SUNDAY
LONG WALK/RUN
80 min: walk 2 min/run 8 min

TOTAL WALK/RUN TIME = 3 HOURS, 22 MINUTES

Recovery Week: For each day above, decrease the amount you walk/run by one-third so that the total walk/run time is 2 hours, 15 minutes.

Course 6

◆ ◆ ◆

MONDAY
Off

TUESDAY
AEROBIC WALK/RUN
40 min: walk 1 min/run 9 min

WEDNESDAY
TEMPO RUN
5-min warm-up **+**

5 x 3 min @ tempo pace with 1-min walk
recovery between reps

+ 5-min cool-down

THURSDAY
Off

FRIDAY
AEROBIC WALK/RUN
50 min: walk 1 min/run 9 min + 4 x 10-sec strides

SATURDAY
Off
or
50-min cross-train

SUNDAY
LONG WALK/RUN
90 min: walk 1 min/run 9 min

TOTAL WALK/RUN TIME = 3 HOURS, 45 MINUTES

Recovery Week: For each day above, decrease the amount you walk/run by one-third so that the total walk/run time is 2 hours, 30 minutes.

RUN YOUR FAT OFF
INTERMEDIATE MENU

Note that some days include more than one menu option. On those days, choose one option from the list.

All Tempo Runs and Aerobic Power Runs are served with a 10-minute warm-up run and 10-minute cool-down run.

Course 1

◆ ◆ ◆

MONDAY
AEROBIC RUN
30 min + 4 x 20-sec strides

TUESDAY
AEROBIC RUN
40 min

WEDNESDAY
TEMPO RUN
10-min warm-up **+**

4 x 5 min @ tempo pace with 1-min rest between reps
or
2 x 10 min @ tempo pace with 2-min rest between reps
or
15 min @ tempo pace

+ 10-min cool-down

THURSDAY
Off

FRIDAY
AEROBIC RUN
30 min + 4 x 20-sec strides

SATURDAY
Off
or
40-min cross-train

SUNDAY
LONG RUN
50 min

TOTAL RUN TIME = 3 HOURS, 30 MINUTES

Recovery Week: For each day above, decrease the amount you run by one-third so that the total run time is 2 hours, 20 minutes.

Course 2

◆ ◆ ◆

MONDAY
AEROBIC RUN
30 min + 4 x 20-sec strides

TUESDAY
AEROBIC RUN
50 min

WEDNESDAY
TEMPO RUN
10-min warm-up **+**

5 x 5 min @ tempo pace with 1-min rest between reps
or
2 x 12 min @ tempo pace with 2-min rest between reps
or
20 min @ tempo pace

+ 10-min cool-down

THURSDAY
Off

FRIDAY
AEROBIC RUN
40 min + 4 x 20-sec strides

SATURDAY
Off
or
50-min cross-train

SUNDAY
LONG RUN
60 min

TOTAL RUN TIME = 4 HOURS, 5 MINUTES

Recovery Week: For each day above, decrease the amount you run by one-third so that the total run time is 2 hours, 43 minutes.

Course 3

◆ ◆ ◆

MONDAY
AEROBIC RUN
40 min + 4 x 20-sec strides

TUESDAY
AEROBIC RUN
60 min

WEDNESDAY
HILL INTERVAL RUN
10-min warm-up **+**

1-min run at 2%, 4%, 6%, 8%, 6%, 4%, 2% grade
with 1-min run recovery between reps at 0% grade
or
1-min run at 2%, 4%, 6%, 8%, 10%, 12%, 14% grade
with 1-min run recovery between reps at 0% grade
or
1-min run at 4%, 8%, 2%, 6%, 3%, 12%, 9% grade
with 1-min run recovery between reps at 0% grade

+ 10-min cool-down

THURSDAY
Off

FRIDAY
AEROBIC RUN
50 min + 4 x 20-sec strides

SATURDAY
Off
or
60-min cross-train

SUNDAY
LONG RUN
70 min

TOTAL RUN TIME = 4 HOURS, 35 MINUTES

Recovery Week: For each day above, decrease the amount you run by one-third so that the total run time is 3 hours, 3 minutes.

Course 4

◆ ◆ ◆

MONDAY
AEROBIC RUN
50 min + 4 x 20-sec strides

TUESDAY
HILL INTERVAL RUN
10-min warm-up +

1-min run at 2%, 4%, 6%, 8%, 6%, 4%, 2% grade
with 1-min run recovery between reps at 0% grade
or
1-min run at 2%, 4%, 6%, 8%, 10%, 12%, 14% grade
with 1-min run recovery between reps at 0% grade
or
1-min run at 4%, 8%, 2%, 6%, 3%, 12%, 9% grade
with 1-min run recovery between reps at 0% grade

+ 10-min cool-down

WEDNESDAY
Off

THURSDAY
AEROBIC RUN
40 min + 4 x 20-sec strides

FRIDAY
TEMPO RUN
10-min warm-up +

6 x 5 min @ tempo pace with 1-min rest between reps
or
3 x 10 min @ tempo pace with 2-min rest between reps
or
25 min @ tempo pace

+ 10-min cool-down

SATURDAY
Off
or
60-min cross-train

SUNDAY
LONG RUN
80 min

TOTAL RUN TIME = 4 HOURS, 55 MINUTES

Recovery Week: For each day above, decrease the amount you run by one-third so that the total run time is 3 hours, 16 minutes.

Course 5

◆ ◆ ◆

MONDAY
AEROBIC RUN
60 min + 4 x 20-sec strides

TUESDAY
AEROBIC POWER RUN
10-min warm-up **+**

4 x 2 min @ hard pace with 2-min jog between reps
or
3 x 3 min @ hard pace with 2-min jog between reps
or
2/3/2/3/2 min @ hard pace with 2-min jog between reps

+ 10-min cool-down

WEDNESDAY
Off

THURSDAY
AEROBIC RUN
50 min + 4 x 20-sec strides

FRIDAY
TEMPO RUN
10-min warm-up **+**

6 x 5 min @ tempo pace with 1-min rest between reps
or
3 x 10 min @ tempo pace with 2-min rest between reps
or
25 min @ tempo pace

+ 10-min cool-down

SATURDAY
Off
or
60-min cross-train

SUNDAY
LONG RUN
90 min

TOTAL RUN TIME = 5 HOURS, 20 MINUTES

Recovery Week: For each day above, decrease the amount you run by one-third so that the total run time is 3 hours, 33 minutes.

Course 6

◆ ◆ ◆

MONDAY
AEROBIC RUN
60 min + 4 x 20-sec strides

TUESDAY
AEROBIC POWER RUN
10-min warm-up +

4 x 2 min @ hard pace with 2-min jog between reps
or
3 x 3 min @ hard pace with 2-min jog between reps
or
2/3/2/3/2 min @ hard pace with 2-min jog between reps

+ 10-min cool-down

WEDNESDAY
Off

THURSDAY
AEROBIC RUN
60 min + 4 x 20-sec strides

FRIDAY
TEMPO RUN
10-min warm-up +

6 x 5 min @ tempo pace with 1-min rest between reps
or
3 x 10 min @ tempo pace with 2-min rest between reps
or
25 min @ tempo pace

+ 10-min cool-down

SATURDAY
Off
or
60-min cross-train

SUNDAY
LONG RUN
90 min

TOTAL RUN TIME = 5 HOURS, 30 MINUTES

Recovery Week: For each day above, decrease the amount you run by one-third so that the total run time is 3 hours, 40 minutes.

RUN YOUR FAT OFF
ADVANCED MENU

Note that some days include more than one menu option. On those days, choose one option from the list. All Hill Runs, Tempo Runs, Aerobic Power Runs, and Anaerobic Runs are served with a 10-minute warm-up run and 10-minute cool-down run.

Course 1

◆ ◆ ◆

MONDAY
AEROBIC RUN
a.m.: 30 min + 5 x 20-sec strides / p.m.: 40 min

TUESDAY
HILL INTERVAL RUN
10-min warm-up **+**

2-min run at 2%, 4%, 6%, 8%, 6%, 4%, 2% grade
with 1-min run recovery between reps at 0% grade
or
2-min run at 2%, 4%, 6%, 8%, 10%, 12%, 14% grade
with 1-min run recovery between reps at 0% grade
or
2-min run at 4%, 8%, 2%, 6%, 3%, 12%, 9% grade
with 1-min run recovery between reps at 0% grade

+ 10-min cool-down

WEDNESDAY
Off

THURSDAY
AEROBIC RUN
40 min

FRIDAY
TEMPO RUN
10-min warm-up **+**

6 x 5 min @ tempo pace with 1-min rest between reps
or
3 x 10 min @ tempo pace with 2-min rest between reps
or
25 min @ tempo pace

+ 10-min cool-down

SATURDAY
Off
or
60-min cross-train

SUNDAY
LONG RUN
90 min

TOTAL RUN TIME = 5 HOURS, 30 MINUTES

Recovery Week: For each day above, decrease the amount you run by one-third so that the total run time is 3 hours, 40 minutes.

Course 2

◆ ◆ ◆

MONDAY
AEROBIC RUN
a.m.: 30 min + 5 x 20-sec strides / p.m.: 40 min

TUESDAY
AEROBIC POWER RUN
10-min warm-up **+**

4 x 2 min @ hard pace with 2-min jog between reps
or
3 x 3 min @ hard pace with 2-min jog between reps
or
2/3/2/3/2 min @ hard pace with 2-min jog between reps

+ 10-min cool-down

WEDNESDAY
Off

THURSDAY
AEROBIC RUN
40 min + 5 x 20-sec strides

FRIDAY
TEMPO RUN
10-min warm-up **+**

6 x 5 min @ tempo pace with 1-min rest between reps
or
3 x 10 min @ tempo pace with 2-min rest between reps
or
25 min @ tempo pace

+ 10-min cool-down

SATURDAY
Off
or
60-min cross-train

SUNDAY
LONG RUN
90 min

TOTAL RUN TIME = 5 HOURS, 20 MINUTES

Recovery Week: For each day above, decrease the amount you run by one-third so that the total run time is 3 hours, 33 minutes.

Course 3

◆ ◆ ◆

MONDAY
AEROBIC RUN
a.m.: 30 min + 5 x 20-sec strides / p.m.: 40 min

TUESDAY
AEROBIC POWER RUN
10-min warm-up **+**

4 x 2 min @ hard pace with 2-min jog between reps

or

3 x 3 min @ hard pace with 2-min jog between reps

or

2/3/2/3/2 min @ hard pace with 2-min jog between reps

+ 10-min cool-down

WEDNESDAY
Off

THURSDAY
AEROBIC RUN
50 min + 5 x 20-sec strides

FRIDAY
TEMPO RUN
10-min warm-up **+**

6 x 5 min @ tempo pace with 1-min rest between reps

or

3 x 10 min @ tempo pace with 2-min rest between reps

or

25 min @ tempo pace

+ 10-min cool-down

SATURDAY
Off

or

70-min cross-train

SUNDAY
LONG RUN
90 min

TOTAL RUN TIME = 5 HOURS, 30 MINUTES

Recovery Week: For each day above, decrease the amount you run by one-third so that the total run time is 3 hours, 40 minutes.

Course 4

• • •

MONDAY
AEROBIC RUN
a.m.: 30 min + 5 x 20-sec strides / p.m.: 40 min

TUESDAY
ANAEROBIC RUN
10-min warm-up **+**

8-10 x 30 sec fast with 2-min jog between reps
or
4-8 x 60 sec fast with 3-min jog between reps
or
2-3 sets of 30/60/90 sec fast with 2-min jog
between reps & 5-min jog between sets

+ 10-min cool-down

WEDNESDAY
Off

THURSDAY
AEROBIC RUN
60 min + 5 x 20-sec strides

FRIDAY
TEMPO RUN
10-min warm-up **+**

6 x 5 min @ tempo pace with 1-min rest between reps
or
3 x 10 min @ tempo pace with 2-min rest between reps
or
25 min @ tempo pace

+ 10-min cool-down

SATURDAY
Off
or
70-min cross-train

SUNDAY
LONG RUN
90 min

TOTAL RUN TIME = 5 HOURS, 50 MINUTES

Recovery Week: For each day above, decrease the amount you run by one-third so that the total run time is 3 hours, 53 minutes.

Course 5

◆ ◆ ◆

MONDAY
AEROBIC RUN
a.m.: 30 min + 5 x 20-sec strides / p.m.: 40 min

TUESDAY
ANAEROBIC RUN
10-min warm-up **+**

8-10 x 30 sec fast with 2-min jog between reps
or
4-8 x 60 sec fast with 3-min jog between reps
or
2-3 sets of 30/60/90 sec fast with 2-min jog
between reps & 5-min jog between sets

+ 10-min cool-down

WEDNESDAY
Off

THURSDAY
AEROBIC RUN
60 min + 5 x 20-sec strides

FRIDAY
AEROBIC POWER RUN
10-min warm-up **+**

4 x 2 min @ hard pace with 2-min jog between reps
or
3 x 3 min @ hard pace with 2-min jog between reps
or
2/3/2/3/2 min @ hard pace with 2-min jog between reps

+ 10-min cool-down

SATURDAY
Off
or
70-min cross-train

SUNDAY
LONG RUN
100 min

TOTAL RUN TIME = 5 HOURS, 50 MINUTES

Recovery Week: For each day above, decrease the amount you run
by one-third so that the total run time is 3 hours, 53 minutes.

Course 6

◆ ◆ ◆

MONDAY
AEROBIC RUN
a.m.: 30 min **+** 5 x 20-sec strides / p.m.: 40 min

TUESDAY
ANAEROBIC RUN
10-min warm-up **+**

8-10 x 30 sec fast with 2-min jog between reps
or
4-8 x 60 sec fast with 3-min jog between reps
or
2-3 sets of 30/60/90 sec fast with 2-min jog
between reps + 5-min jog between sets

+ 10-min cool-down

WEDNESDAY
Off

THURSDAY
AEROBIC RUN
60 min + 5 x 20-sec strides

FRIDAY
ANAEROBIC RUN
10-min warm-up **+**

8-10 x 30 sec fast with 2-min jog between reps
or
4-8 x 60 sec fast with 3-min jog between reps
or
2-3 sets of 30/60/90 sec fast with 2-min jog between reps
+ 5-min jog between sets

+ 10-min cool-down

SATURDAY
Off
or
70-min cross-train

SUNDAY
LONG RUN
110 min

TOTAL RUN TIME = 6 HOURS

Recovery Week: For each day above, decrease the amount you run by one-third so that the total run time is 4 hours.

The Run Your Fat Off Menu Recipes

Warm-Ups

    1 pair running shoes
    1 or more running buddies (optional)
    1 iPod with your favorite songs (optional)

Run (or walk/run) for the prescribed amount of time at a comfortable pace. To create a smooth transition between warm-up and workout, warm-up should get progressively faster until you reach the pace at which you'll run during the workout.

Cool-Downs

    1 pair running shoes
    1 or more running buddies (optional)
    1 iPod with your favorite songs (optional)

Run (or walk/run) for the prescribed amount of time at a comfortable pace.

Aerobic Runs

    1 pair running shoes
    1 or more running buddies (optional)
    1 iPod with your favorite songs (optional)

Run at an easy, gentle pace, making sure to run slowly enough to complete the prescribed amount of time. The speed isn't as important as the duration because the goal is to build endurance and burn calories. The easier your aerobic runs, the more running you can handle each week. If you're a new runner, mix walking and running to make the workouts more manageable. In this case, walk at a brisk pace—fast enough that you feel you're walking fast, yet slowly enough that it's not a run. As you adapt to running and build your endurance, you'll find that you can run longer before taking a walking break. With every accumulated minute you run or run/walk, you're burning calories and improving your endurance.

To gradually and carefully run more miles, start with however much you are currently running and run the same total weekly distance (or time) for 2 weeks (or more if you need to). Next, increase the mileage by adding 1 mile (or add 5 to 10 minutes) to each of your runs for a week. Then back off by about one-third of that total weekly mileage or time for one recovery week. Continue to add miles (or time) in the same fashion. For example, if you run 3 days per week, your weekly mileage progression can look like this:

Weeks 1 to 4: 5-5-8-5 miles per week

Weeks 5 to 8: 8-8-11-7 miles per week

Weeks 9 to 12: 11-11-14-9 miles per week

In other words, run 5 miles in week 1, 5 miles again in week 2, increase to 8 miles (by adding 1 mile per day to each of the 3 days) in week 3, and reduce to 5 miles in week 4 to recover. Continue the same pattern in weeks 5 through 8 and 9 through 12.

If that's too slow of a progression for you, no problem. You can progress faster, still by adding 1 mile (or by adding 5 to 10 minutes) to each day you run each week for 3 weeks before cutting back for a recovery week. Using the example of three runs per week:

Weeks 1 to 4: 5-8-11-7 miles per week
Weeks 5 to 8: 11-14-17-11 miles per week
Weeks 9 to 12: 17-20-23-15 miles per week

There really is no rule regarding how much you run or walk/run, only that you pick a starting point that is right for you and progress gradually to enable your body (and mind) to adapt.

Long Runs

1 pair running shoes
1 sense of adventure
1 or more running buddies (optional)
1 iPod with your favorite songs (optional)

Run at an easy, gentle pace, making sure to run slow enough to complete the prescribed amount of time. Long runs are one case in which slower is better. Because your legs have little concept of distance, only of intensity and time, the amount of time you spend on your feet is more important than the number of miles you cover. As you become a runner, you'll notice that runners are creatures of habit and are obsessed with miles, but time is what really matters.

Tempo Runs

1 pair running shoes
Your A game
1 iPod with your favorite songs (optional)

Preheat and prepare your body with a 10-minute easy warm-up. For this workout, which gives your aerobic system a boost that takes you to your aerobic steady-state running limit, run at as steady a pace as possible for the amount of time prescribed. Don't try to do each tempo run faster than the one you did last week; instead, try to increase the amount of time you hold the pace (as directed in the *Run Your Fat Off* menus).

Run at tempo pace for the specified amount of time, with short rest intervals. Run each rep at exactly the same pace. By breaking the continuous tempo run into shorter segments with rest intervals, you can run more total time or distance at tempo pace in a single workout. The pace should feel comfortably hard and at the upper end of being purely aerobic—a 7 to 8 on a scale of 1 to 10 of perceived effort, with 10 being as hard as you can run. For the recovery intervals, walk around a bit between each rep. If you do the workouts on a treadmill, decrease the speed to a slow walk to recover before increasing the treadmill speed for the next rep. If you have run a race before, tempo pace can be determined from race pace:

For beginner and recreational/intermediate runners:
◆ About 10 to 15 seconds per mile slower than 5K race pace
◆ Equal or very close to 10K race pace (if you run slower than 53 minutes for 10K, your tempo pace will be slightly faster than 10K race pace)
◆ 80 to 85 percent max heart rate (see the box on page 9 to learn how to determine your maximum heart rate)

For competitive, trained runners:
◆ About 25 to 30 seconds per mile slower than 5K race pace

◆ About 15 to 20 seconds per mile slower than 10K race pace
◆ 85 to 90 percent max heart rate

If you have never run a race before, run by effort at a 7 to 8 on a scale of 1 to 10 and by heart rate (if you have a heart rate monitor) using the guidelines above. Monitor your breathing—if you're breathing to the point at which you feel out of breath, you're running too fast.

Aerobic Power Runs

1 pair running shoes
Your A game
1 iPod with your favorite songs (optional)

Preheat and prepare your body with a 10-minute easy warm-up followed by a few 10-second strides at a fast but controlled pace. For the best cardiovascular workout on the planet, alternate hard running for 3 to 5 minutes at or near your maximum heart rate with slow jogging for the same amount of time or slightly less than the amount of time as you run to catch your breath and keep your aerobic engine running. The active recovery jogs help your heart rate get higher earlier in the next running period so you can spend more time running at close to your max heart rate. If you're too fatigued to jog, then walk briskly.

Aerobic power runs should feel hard but manageable. They're hard because you're working at your heart's maximum capability to do its job (pump blood and oxygen), but not so hard that you can't complete another rep. Base the workouts off of heart rate and/or effort, reaching 95 to

100 percent of your max heart rate and a 9 on a scale of 1 to 10 during each period of running.

Make the running periods at least a couple of minutes; running for less time doesn't give your heart rate enough time to get high enough to acquire the cardiovascular benefit of the workout. As you progress, cap the running periods at 4 to 5 minutes; running hard for longer prevents you from repeating the running period more than a couple of times in one workout.

Make aerobic power runs more challenging by altering the components of the workouts. In order of difficulty from hardest to easiest, make the interval workouts harder by (1) increasing the duration of each running period, (2) increasing the number of repetitions, or (3) decreasing the duration of the recovery intervals.

Anaerobic Runs

1 pair running shoes

Your A game

Preheat and prepare your body with a 10-minute easy warm-up followed by a few 10-second strides at a fast but controlled pace. For this workout, which develops powerful muscles and unleashes your inner sprinter, run fast enough for the prescribed amount of time so that you feel like you're sprinting, but not so fast that you can't repeat the sprint after a short recovery. Run tall and swing your arms from your shoulders in a fast and controlled manner. Imagine grabbing the ground or treadmill belt with the ball of your foot, like a cat pawing the ground, and pushing the ground behind you.

Hill Runs

1 pair running shoes

1 outdoor hill or treadmill

Your A game

1 iPod with your favorite songs (optional)

Preheat and prepare your body with a 10-minute easy warm-up followed by a few 10-second strides at a fast but controlled pace. For this heart-thumping workout, which burns a lot of calories as you work against gravity, run up the hill for the prescribed amount of time. Use your arms and lean from your ankles into the hill. If outside, find a fairly steep hill and jog or walk down the hill to recover. If on a treadmill, lower the grade to 0% to recover.

Strides

1 pair running shoes

1 or more running buddies (optional)

After completing your aerobic run or walk/run, run a series of controlled sprints for the prescribed amount of time, taking full recovery (about 2 minutes) between each rep. Don't sprint all out; the sprints should feel fast but relaxed. Focus on your running technique.

Cross-Training

Cardio equipment of choice

1 gym or swimming pool

1 iPod with your favorite songs (optional)

Cross-train with one of the following activities for the prescribed amount of time or take a group fitness or yoga class at the gym.

Elliptical Trainer: One of the most popular pieces of cardio equipment in the gym, the elliptical trainer most closely resembles the movement of running without the impact, and it's still weight bearing.

Water Running: Running in deep water is a great opportunity to run without impact. The resistance from the water offers a great workout. You can water run with or without a flotation vest (such as an AquaJogger) for buoyancy. Although this is a great cross-training activity for your legs, your heart rate doesn't rise as high when in the water.

Cross-Country Skiing Machine: Only one activity improves aerobic fitness more than running—cross-country skiing. If you don't have access to snow or ski equipment, try a cross-country skiing machine in the gym, like a NordicTrack. Although it takes some time to learn the skill, it's a great cross-training activity that burns tons of calories and raises heart rate.

Swimming: Swimming is a great activity to train your upper body muscles, which are often neglected in runners. Swimming also gives your legs a break from the pounding. If you have poor posture and a weak upper body, you can swim to work on upper body postural muscles and increase upper body strength.

Cycling: Cycling is another no-impact activity that gives you a break from running while still giving you a great workout for your legs. It's a great way to develop leg power, although there's less range of motion when compared to running. Use a stationary bike in the gym or take a high-intensity Spinning class.

Rowing Machine: Rowing is a great whole-body, no-impact, cross-training activity. It makes you cardiovascularly fit, and it works the upper and lower body at the same time, although the power of the stroke comes mainly from your legs. To get the most out of rowing, you first have to learn proper technique, which includes pushing with your legs before pulling with your arms.

Yoga: I confess that I don't really understand the appeal of yoga. As a runner, I find yoga too stationary, with the effort concentrated on specific muscles and postures. But yoga is great for flexibility, balance, and strength, although it doesn't burn a lot of calories. And its meditative component enhances breathing and focus. For a more athletic yoga workout, choose the Ashtanga or Vinyasa versions.

◆ ◆ ◆ ◆ ◆

"I THOUGHT, 'WHY NOT?'" Roger Leszczynski says about the flyer he saw at the YMCA for an upcoming 5K. "I wanted to see what I could do." From that first 5K, he was hooked on running races. "I set goals to improve my time and fitness by comparing my results to people who looked similar to me."

One day, there was a marathon in Roger's town. He decided to watch, and he noticed that some good runners weren't as pencil thin as he had expected. So he decided the next year he would run it himself. Wanting more of an outdoor lifestyle, he moved from Connecticut to San Diego "because of the sun," he says. "I wanted to be outdoors all the time."

Living in San Diego, the birthplace of the triathlon, he added cycling and swimming to his running. And he started competing.

"Triathlons helped me overcome a fear of swimming and enabled me to continue aerobic training without burning out," he says. Roger has completed every triathlon distance, from sprint triathlons to an Ironman, which includes a 2.2-mile ocean swim, 112-mile bike, and 26.2-mile marathon run with no rest in between. "I still respect the short distances," he says. "Those races can hurt!" Making it down to 160 pounds, he also ran a 2:59 marathon to qualify for the prestigious Boston Marathon, where he ran 2:54, a respectable time for anyone, much less someone who used to be 260 pounds and ate pizzas for lunch.

Roger didn't enter that first 5K race so he could lose weight; he ran the race because "I wanted to see what I could do."

Having adopted an active lifestyle, Roger recognized that sitting at a desk all day as a software engineer was bad for his

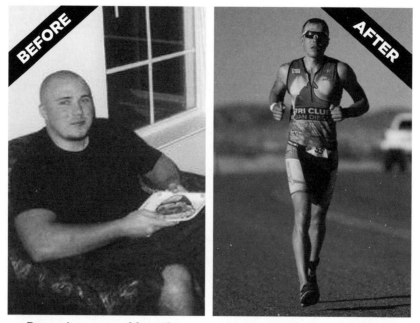

Roger Leszczynski, eating pizzas at 260 pounds.

Leszczynski now, competing in triathlons at 160 pounds.

health. He decided to take a large pay cut and become a bike messenger, delivering documents between law offices and courts. He also helps to run SD Bike Commuter, a unique program that promotes exercise and the "green" movement by partnering with local businesses in San Diego to offer discounts and rewards to people who bike to those businesses.

"Education was key," he says. "There was a lot of trial and error, such as silly low-fat diets. It was an opportunity to learn nutrition, biochemistry, even politics—how big companies prefer to profit at the cost of our health."

When I asked him about his weight-loss journey, he says, "Losing weight is an absolute mental challenge. Instant gratification isn't the way. It was a long process—4 years to be 100 pounds less. Sacrifices were needed, but eventually my taste buds became reprogrammed so that I didn't crave heavily processed foods anymore. Carrots now satisfy me more than potato chips."

CHAPTER 5

Running Nutrition

"I LEARNED HOW EASY ANOREXIC-TYPE THOUGHTS CAN OCCUR."

NESTLED AT THE JUNCTION of the Kansas River and Big Blue River in Kansas's northeastern town of Manhattan sits the campus of Kansas State University. Inside the university's Justin Hall is the Department of Food, Nutrition, Dietetics and Health, where 47-year-old department head Dr. Mark Haub sits at his desk, looking over the manuscript of his latest study on the effects of physical activity on the fermentation of resistant starch—carbohydrate that is resistant to digestion and absorption in the small intestine and is instead fermented in the large intestine, much like fiber. He and his research team carry out detailed experiments to determine the efficacy of foods, ingredients, and supplements on metabolic outcomes, primarily diabetes and obesity. His current research focuses on how dietary carbohydrate, fiber, and whole grains affect glucose metabolism and gut health. To determine this, he and his graduate students feed volunteers barley, brown rice, and a combination of barley and brown rice. After the different meals are consumed, they take numerous blood samples to measure glucose, insulin, cholesterol, and markers of inflammation, and they analyze the volunteers' fecal samples for their microorganisms.

An important facet of Mark's research is the unique contribution of fiber to health and how fiber can be integrated into the food supply in a manner that people will be willing to purchase and consume it. As part of his research, one of the key questions he and his students hope to answer is whether lifestyle (i.e., physical activity) determines our health and *microbiome*—the collection of microorganisms that resides in our bodies, creating their own ecological community—or if our microbiome determines our health more than does our lifestyle.

Before his days of being a university professor and scientist, Mark ran 80 to 85 miles per week, often running twice per day. He ran cross-country and track in high school in Kansas and in college at Fort Hays State University. After college, he ran two marathons, including the 2000 Boston Marathon in a time of 2:54.

After completing a postdoctoral research position in Arkansas, Mark moved back to Kansas to pursue a career in academia, and running took a backseat. "I became focused on work and exercised more leisurely," he says. He started as an assistant professor, acquired tenure, and worked his way up to become department head. In 2004, he and his wife became parents and his focus shifted to parenthood. And he gained weight.

In 2010, Mark was borderline obese at 201 pounds and a BMI of nearly 29. "According to many people, I had weight to lose," he says. "The USDA guidelines were also about to come out, and one of the drafts stated that refined grain foods, solid fats, and added sugars are obesogenic. If foods are obesogenic, then I should gain weight eating mostly those foods regardless of the caloric intake or caloric balance." But, he reasoned, if pure calorie counting—calories in versus calories out—is what matters most for weight loss, rather than the nutritional value of the food, then it shouldn't matter what foods are eaten, as long as he eats fewer calories than he expends. And so a professor's class project was born.

◆ ◆ ◆ ◆ ◆

GROWING UP, my twin brother was a big fan of Twinkies. Me, not so much. I could take them or leave them. I was always more a fan of sugar cereals. Cinnamon Toast Crunch was my favorite. As an adult, I like bananas. A lot. I eat one almost every day. It's a good thing that bananas are high in carbohydrate, potassium, magnesium, vitamin B_6, and fiber, all nutrients that are good for runners. I also like apple juice, even more than bananas. "Apple juice" were my first words as a baby. Seriously. I said "apple juice" even before I said "Mom" or "Dad." Unfortunately, apple juice is not as healthy as bananas are, but the sugar in apple juice provides my muscles with a quick source of energy to run.

People who want to lose weight always ask me how often they should run. I usually respond, "You only have to run on the days you eat." (Not everyone gets my sense of humor.) This chapter is all about eating.

I admit I have always eaten what and how much I want, and I have never tracked the calories I consume, perhaps because I know I'm going to run off any excess calories anyway. I have never tried or needed to lose weight. But I have also never *gained* weight, which underscores the importance of daily running for maintaining weight. It turns out that when you are very physically active, hunger is an excellent regulator of body weight. I eat only when I'm hungry and just enough to satisfy my hunger. I have been running 6 days per week since I was in sixth grade, including plenty of high-intensity interval training and races and, at age 44, my weight is exactly the same as it was when I was in high school. (Don't hate me!) Running is the best fat-burning torch there is. But running, despite its large calorie burn, is also not enough if I want to *lose* weight. And just because I run a lot doesn't mean I should eat Froot Loops.

What? Wait a minute! Did Dr. Jason just say that running won't make you lose weight? No, I didn't exactly say that. Running can help you lose weight because, as you'll experience, it burns more calories than just about anything else. But burning calories is only half the equation when it comes to weight loss. Exercise by itself frequently does not lead to weight loss. With all of the gyms and personal trainers and fitness gadgets on the market, the rate of obesity is still rising. Many people exercise and still don't lose weight. Why?

It takes a *lot* of running—and therefore a lot of effort and time—to accomplish the caloric deficit needed to lose a significant amount of weight. And, although more running burns more calories than any other exercise and shifts your metabolism toward a greater reliance on fat, your body is very smart. At high levels of physical activity, your body adjusts the number of calories it expends the rest of the day to keep your total daily caloric expenditure within a narrow range.

Running, like any aerobic exercise, also increases hunger. People tend to eat more when they run more to compensate for the calories they've expended, so their weight stays the same, no matter what that weight is. That's why my weight has not changed since high school. It's also why overweight people have a hard time losing weight even when they start running. Research as far back as 1956 published in the *American Journal of Clinical Nutrition* showed that people's caloric intake increases the more active they are. But the converse is not true. Below a specific level of activity—what the scientists called the "sedentary zone"—a decrease in activity is not followed by a matched decrease in food intake but rather by an increase. Thus, people at the extreme ends of physical activity—those who exercise a lot and those who don't exercise at all—are the ones who eat the most.

Many runners, myself included, look forward to treating themselves to a big meal or a fancy smoothie after a long run. The thought of a big plate of pancakes with boysenberry syrup and a chocolate banana smoothie is often enough to get me through another few miles of a long run. But if you want to lose weight, you can't treat yourself with excess calories after your runs. You can have some, perhaps a few forkfuls of pancakes and a few sips of the smoothie, but not so much that you negate the calories you just burned

> **"TOO MANY PEOPLE OVERCOMPENSATE WITH CALORIES AFTER THEIR RUNS, THINKING THAT 'THEY EARNED IT.'"**

on the run. Too many people overcompensate with calories after their runs, thinking that "they earned it." And if you don't run every day—which is the case for nearly all beginning runners—that leaves the door open for too many uncompensated calories on the days you're not running.

To lose weight, you must accept hunger as a necessary side effect. You have to cut back on the number of calories you eat and drink, despite exercising more, which means you're going to be hungry. The good news is, because of its effect on mitochondria and the muscles' capacity to burn fat, chronic running increases fat metabolism more than it increases appetite.

It is much easier, both theoretically and practically, to consume fewer calories by changing one's diet than to burn more calories by running more. For example, it may take you about 30 minutes to run 3 miles and burn 300 calories, but it takes you no time at all to decide not to eat a 300-calorie blueberry muffin.

What this means is that a combined running-and-diet approach is significantly more effective for weight loss than either approach alone. There have been hundreds of studies that have shown this. On the *Run Your Fat Off* plan, your nutrition plan needs to steer as many calories as possible into meeting your running-induced metabolic needs rather than into fat storage. You need to consume enough calories to fuel your running, maintain your resting metabolic rate, and meet the recommended daily intake for all the essential nutrients, but less than what you expend through running and other exercise.

CALORIE RESTRICTION

For this idea of eating less, we must thank Luigi Cornaro, a fifthteenth-century Italian nobleman who adopted a calorie-restricted diet at age 35 to address his failing health. His popular book, *Discorsi della vita sobria* (*Discourses on the Temperate Life*), describes his diet, which consisted of just 350 grams (about 1,500 to 1,600 calories) of food per day (including bread, egg yolk, meat, and soup) and, interestingly enough, 414 milliliters (nearly three glasses) of wine. (For comparison, one slice of white bread has 80 calories and modern-day food labels are based on 2,000 calories per day.) It worked. The diet cured him of his ailments, including gout, stomach pain, and fever, in less than a year, and he went on to live to 102 years old.

It wasn't until early in the twentieth century that scientific research caught up with Luigi Cornaro. In longitudinal experiments on rats done in the 1930s, scientists found that rats fed 30 to 60 percent fewer calories grew at a much slower rate and lived nearly twice as long as rats that were fed more. Since then, many studies over the last 85 years have shown that, from

rodents to primates, caloric restriction extends lifespan and protects against the deterioration of biological functions, delaying
or reducing the risk of many age-related diseases. And the term
caloric restriction was born.

Furthermore, the large body of research has shown that
low-calorie diets (about 1,000 to 1,200 calories per day) can reduce total body weight by an average of 8 percent over 3 to 12
months. If you weigh 200 pounds, that's 16 pounds lost. Very
low-calorie diets (about 400 to 500 calories per day) produce
greater initial weight loss than low-calorie diets, but the long-
term (more than 1 year) weight loss is not different from that of
low-calorie diets. I don't recommend diets as low as 400 to 500
calories since it won't give you enough energy to run. Eating so
few calories will also deprive you of the essential nutrients you
need to maintain your health, and it is too far below your resting
metabolic rate.

Is it tough to eat less in our current obesogenic environment of
fast, cheap, high-calorie food? You bet it is. There are more than
14,300 McDonald's restaurants in the United States and more
than 35,000 worldwide. And McDonald's, of course, is not the only
culprit. Cheap, non-nutritious food is everywhere. But running
has the power to influence your eating habits.

Take, for example, a study from the University of Florida's medical school, where scientists did a series of experiments during
which they accommodated rats to a diet of either normal chow
food (17 percent fat, 58 percent carbohydrate, 25 percent protein) or high-fat food (60 percent fat, 20 percent carbohydrate,
20 percent protein). The rats were then placed in a cage with running wheels. After a week, the running wheels were taken away,
and the rats were given both meal options from which to choose.
The scientists found that in the absence of running wheels, the
rats hardly touched the nutritious low-fat chow food, instead

opting for the high-fat food. In contrast, when the rats had free access to running wheels, they consumed much less of the high-fat food. This was true for both the rats who had been accustomed to the high-fat food and those that had been eating the normal chow food. The access to running wheels reduced the rats' preference for the high-fat meal. Although you're a human and not a rat, it's possible, and even probable, that if you don't exercise, you're more likely to consume a high-fat diet than if you do exercise, partly because you're more likely to engage in unhealthy behaviors when you're not physically active, and vice versa.

> **" NOT ONLY ARE YOU MORE LIKELY TO EAT HEALTHIER IF YOU RUN, YOU CAN ALSO OUTRUN A BAD DIET, OR AT LEAST DIMINISH ITS EFFECTS."**

Not only are you more likely to eat healthier if you run, you can also outrun a bad diet, or at least diminish its effects. To prove that, we return to the National Runners' and Walkers' Health Studies. In one of the studies, researchers analyzed data from 106,737 runners to determine the relationship between how much meat and fruit they ate and their body mass index (BMI) and chest and hip circumferences. Normally, BMI (along with body weight) tends to increase in association with greater meat and lesser fruit consumption. But it turned out that running diminished the association of BMI with higher meat and lower fruit consumption. And the effect of running was dose dependent: The more miles people ran per week, the lower the association. In both men and women who ran at least 5 miles (8 kilometers) per day, eating meat was much less associated with their BMI and chest and hip circumferences when compared to those who ran less than 1.25 miles (2 kilo-meters) per day. And running at least 5 miles per day offset the downside of not eating fruit even more. One of the reasons why running diminishes the negative impact of eating more meat and less fruit is that running improves your ability to use fat, both when you run and during the rest of the day. If you constantly use fat (and carbohydrate) to fuel your running, it doesn't settle on your body.

MACRONUTRIENT COMPOSITION OF THE RUNNING DIET

Although the number of daily calories is the most important char-acteristic of the *Run Your Fat Off* plan, the nutritional composition of your diet also matters for health and running performance. The type of calories you consume can also affect the quantity of calories you consume.

Carbohydrate

Carbohydrate is a runner's best friend. To find out why, we have to go way back—all the way back to the time life on Earth began. A long time ago, before you and I were born, the atmosphere of primitive Earth was thought to have been made up of hydrogen and contained little or no oxygen. So the earliest organisms on Earth had to develop an anaerobic (non-oxygen-using) way of producing energy. Since carbohydrate can be broken down with-out oxygen, organisms relied on carbohydrate. All these millions of years later, carbohydrate is still muscles' fuel of choice.

When your muscles run out of carbohydrate, they don't per-form well, and your running pace dramatically slows. Muscles re-spond to the low carbohydrate tank by synthesizing and storing more than what had previously been present, a process largely controlled by the hormone insulin. Like your muscles, brain function is also impaired by a lack of carbohydrate. If you don't have enough carbs, you literally can't think straight and your reasoning skills diminish. In order to work out at a high intensity, prevent hypoglycemia (low blood sugar) during your runs, refuel your muscles, and strengthen your immune system, you need to eat enough carbs. Over many months and years of running, your muscles will become better at using fat for energy during slower runs, but you need carbs, especially when you first start running. Your body's store of carbohydrate is relatively limited and can be acutely manipulated on a daily basis by your dietary intake or even by a single run.

Despite what the media may want you to believe, sugar is not inherently bad. When you consume carbohydrate, the concentration of insulin in your blood rises, which triggers the transportation of that carbohydrate (glucose) from your blood into your cells. It is then that glucose's fate is determined. If you eat more carbohydrate than your body needs for energy, which is easy to do when you eat a lot of sugar, the excess glucose is either stored as glycogen in your muscles and liver or as body fat. As I explained in Chapter 2, which of those two fates is chosen depends on how full your glycogen stores are, which depends on how much you run. Running uses sugar for energy. The amount of carbohydrate you consume should fluctuate in accordance with how much you run—the more you run, the more carbohydrate you need. During the weeks you run less, consume less carbohydrate. I have a friend who used to run 100 miles per week as he trained for the U.S. Olympic Marathon Trials, and he liked to tell me how he would eat a pound of pasta in one sitting. He was 6 feet and 150 pounds. Obviously, his body needed a lot of carbohydrate to support his training.

Although all carbohydrate can fuel your running, not all carbohydrate contributes equally to a nutritional diet. Quickly digestible, high-glycemic carbohydrate (simple sugars), such as fruit juice, honey, molasses, dairy, soda, and sweets, raises your blood sugar to provide energy, is often low in essential vitamins and minerals, and, in the case of desserts, is often high in fat. High-glycemic carbohydrate is also associated with an increased risk of obesity. Low-glycemic carbohydrate, such as whole-grain breads and cereals, rice, pasta, fruits, vegetables, and yogurt, doesn't raise your blood sugar nearly as much, is more nutrient dense, and is rich in fiber. Try to limit high-glycemic carbohydrate for immediately after running and consume low-glycemic carbohydrate the rest of the day. Your metabolism converts all types of carbohydrate into glucose because that is the fuel you use; however, if you consume too much, it will get stored as fat.

Many studies have shown that decreasing the carbohydrate content of your diet to under 50 percent to as low as 4 percent of daily calories—especially the high-glycemic variety (i.e., sugar)—can lead to rapid weight loss. A low-carb diet means low blood glucose, which stimulates the breakdown of fat. Drastically reducing carbohydrate intake also improves metabolic health in people with insulin resistance, type 2 diabetes, high total cholesterol and LDL ("bad") cholesterol, and low HDL ("good") cholesterol level. Low-carbohydrate diets became popular because they worked, at least in the short term. But remember that you can't run at a high intensity without carbohydrate. So, consume less carbohydrate in order to lose weight, but still enough to support your running (about 40 to 50 percent of total daily calories).

Protein

Growing up in New York City, I walked under a lot of scaffolding. There's always construction in New York. Damaged buildings are being repaired, new buildings are being built. The construction never ends.

When you run, construction inside your body also never ends. Your body is an architectural masterpiece comprised of protein. The protein you eat is broken down into amino acids, the metaphorical bricks that are used to (1) repair your muscles of the microscopic damage they incur from your running workouts; (2) build new functional proteins and cells that make you fitter and healthier, like mitochondria, enzymes, red blood cells, and antibodies; and (3) build transport proteins that move molecules from one place to another, like the protein albumin, which transports fatty acids to your muscles and liver for oxidation when your blood sugar is low. Every time you run, a strong signal is sent to construct the scaffolding and get busy building proteins.

The amino acids from the protein you eat are so busy being used to build proteins that they can't supply energy for running itself, leaving that responsibility to carbohydrate and fat. Protein normally contributes only about 5 percent of your running fuel, but if your muscle glycogen stores are low, protein will be asked to pick up the slack and can contribute up to 15 percent of the energy used. Thus, to prevent your muscles from relying on protein when you run, they need to have enough carbohydrate available.

One of the benefits of eating protein is that it makes you feel fuller and thus can help to control your appetite. If you lack protein in your diet, not only are you likely to feel hungry more often, you are more likely to experience decreased muscle mass, a suppressed immune system, increased risk of injury, and chronic fatigue. Runners at risk of insufficient protein intake include those on a very low-calorie or vegetarian or vegan diet; low-calorie diets put all nutrients at risk for being insufficient, and plant proteins are less well digested than are animal proteins. A well-balanced vegetarian or vegan diet can supply enough protein as long as the protein sources are varied and enough calories are consumed during the day.

Research has shown that diets containing 0.4 gram of protein per pound of body weight (0.8 gram per kilogram) per day are effective for weight and fat loss when cutting calories to lose weight. For a 200-pound person, this is 80 grams of protein eaten throughout the day, which is equivalent to a 10- to 11-ounce steak.

Fat

Along with carbohydrate, fat is a popular scapegoat for making people fat and has therefore become a prominent topic in weight-loss conversations. It's our brains' fault. Perhaps the most significant evolutionary change in the modern human was growth of the brain, from 850 to 1,200 cubic centimeters as *Homo erectus* (between 1.5 million and 130,000 years ago) to 1,350 to 1,400 cubic centimeters as *Homo sapiens* (first showing up 130,000 years ago).

The brain is your body's Ferrari—it's an expensive organ to maintain. Humans expend a much larger share of their resting energy budget on brain metabolism than do other primates or non-primate mammals. Where do we get the energy to support our brains? From high-energy fat. Research on the diets of primates shows that the high cost of a large human brain is supported by diets that are rich in fat. Greater brain size also appears to have consequences for human body composition, particularly when we are young. Human infants have more body fat than do the infants of other mammals, which enables human brains to grow by having a ready supply of stored energy. Interestingly, when dietary fat is not readily available, human infants and toddlers preserve their body fat by stunting their body's linear growth and even increase the amount of fat they store so the brain has enough for itself. From an evolutionary perspective, the increased consumption of fat—and thus the energy that comes with it—appears to have been necessary for promoting brain growth in humans.

Because fat supplies more than twice the number of calories

per gram when compared to carbohydrate and protein, it provides a concentrated calorie source to give you energy. Fat also helps to produce hormones, is an important component of cell membranes, contributes to nerve function, and carries the fat-soluble vitamins A, D, E, and K into your body.

The earliest weight-loss diets of the 1970s relied on cutting fat. Eating fat, they reasoned, made you fat. Sounds logical. However, fat *per se* doesn't make you fat. Because fat has 9 calories per gram versus 4 for carbohydrate and protein, the extra calories you get from a high-fat diet are what make you fat. Low-fat diets are no better than calorie-restricted diets in achieving long-term weight loss in overweight or obese people. A diet too low in fat, common among individuals trying to lose weight, limits running performance by inhibiting the storage of fat inside your muscles, which can cause premature fatigue during your runs (when you run slowly, muscles rely on fat that is stored inside them). So you need enough fat to run and to meet fat's other responsibilities (maintenance of cell membrane integrity, hormone production, and the absorption of fat-soluble vitamins), but not too much that you clog your arteries and have a heart attack.

There are three kinds of fat: saturated, polyunsaturated, and monounsaturated. Saturated fat has a negative effect on your blood cholesterol level and can increase your chances of developing heart disease. (Trans fats, which are the result of the commercial process of hydrogenation, behave just like saturated fat in your body, increasing your risk for heart disease.) Try to limit the amount of saturated fat that you eat. All animal products, such as meat, poultry, cheese, and whole milk contain saturated fat, which is solid at room temperature. Butter; lard; tropical oils such as palm, coconut, and palm kernel oil; and hydrogenated fat found in margarine, commercial baked goods, and snack foods also contain saturated and trans fat.

Polyunsaturated fat, such as soybean oil and sunflower oil, and monounsaturated fat, such as peanut oil and olive oil, are liquid at room temperature and have a positive effect on your blood cholesterol level and heart health. To lose weight, choose monounsaturated or polyunsaturated fat over saturated fat. Consuming saturated fat results in less fat being burned and more fat being stored when compared to consuming unsaturated fat. Diets high in unsaturated fat induce more weight loss than do diets high in saturated fat. Bottom line: Unsaturated fat is good for weight loss and health, saturated fat is bad for both.

WHICH MACRONUTRIENTS ARE BEST FOR WEIGHT LOSS?

Walk up and down the weight-loss aisle of any bookstore, and you'll quickly learn that there is intense debate about the type of diet that is most effective for weight loss—low-carb, high-carb, low-fat, high-fat, high-protein. Food composition has become unnecessarily very complex. We have an entire society so infatuated with the nutrients of food that we have lost sight of food itself.

To determine what the composition of your diet should look, or rather taste, like, a number of studies have examined the effectiveness of the macronutrient distribution of popular diets on weight loss. These studies have shown that macronutrient combination doesn't matter much. Take, for example, a study from the Harvard School of Public Health, published in the prestigious *New England Journal of Medicine* in 2009, in which scientists randomly assigned 811 overweight adults to one of the following four diets for 2 years:

1. a low-fat, average-protein, high-carb diet (20 percent fat, 15 percent protein, 65 percent carbohydrate)
2. a low-fat, high-protein, average-carb diet (20 percent fat, 25 percent protein, 55 percent carbohydrate)

3. a high-fat, average-protein, average-carb diet (40 percent fat, 15 percent protein, 45 percent carbohydrate)

4. a high-fat, high-protein, low-carb diet (40 percent fat, 25 percent protein, 35 percent carbohydrate)

After 6 months, the participants assigned to each diet had lost an average of 13 pounds. After 12 months, they began to regain some of the weight. After 2 years, the number of pounds lost remained similar in those who were assigned to a diet with 15 percent protein (6.6 pounds) and 25 percent protein (7.9 pounds); in those assigned to a diet with 20 percent fat (7.3 pounds) and 40 percent fat (7.3 pounds); and in those assigned to a diet with 65 percent carbohydrate (6.4 pounds) and 35 percent carbohydrate (7.5 pounds). For weight loss, it doesn't seem to matter what the precise macronutrient combination of the diet is.

In another study, scientists at the Basel Institute for Clinical Epidemiology in Basel, Switzerland, analyzed randomized-controlled studies comparing the effect of low-carbohydrate diets without caloric restriction to calorie-restricted, low-fat diets in overweight individuals with a BMI of at least 25. They found that low-carbohydrate diets were more effective for weight loss after 6 months. After 12 months, however, the weight loss from the low-carb diets was no different than that from the low-fat diets. Whether you reduce carbs or fat, you lose weight because you inevitably consume fewer calories.

In another study published in the *Journal of the American Dietetic Association*, scientists from the Beltsville Human Nutrition Research Center, one of the laboratories of the U.S. Department of Agriculture's Agricultural Research Service, examined the relationship between nine popular diets and diet quality, which included data from 10,014 adults. They found that the lowest caloric intake occurred on a vegetarian diet. Diet quality was highest for the diet that was high in carbohydrate and included at least one serving from the five major food groups in the USDA Food Guide Pyramid. It was lowest for the low-carbohydrate diet, likely because low-carb diets lack fruits and vegetables. Body mass index (BMI) was significantly lower for men and women on a vegetarian diet and on a high-carbohydrate diet, while the highest BMI belonged to those on a low-carbohydrate diet. Perhaps this is due to the fact that you can run more and at a higher intensity when you consume a high-carbohydrate diet, and more and higher-intensity running helps you lose weight and gives you a lower BMI.

" WEIGHT LOSS IS INDEPENDENT OF DIET COMPOSITION AND CALORIC RESTRICTION IS THE KEY VARIABLE ASSOCIATED WITH WEIGHT REDUCTION."

From their review of more than 200 other studies that examined diets of different macronutrient compositions, the scientists found that weight loss is independent of diet composition and that caloric restriction is the key variable associated with weight reduction, at least for the short-term nature of most studies.

What about after you have lost weight? Does the macronutrient composition of your diet matter then? To answer this question, scientists at the University of Copenhagen in Denmark compared the effects of three different diets on the maintenance of at least 8 percent weight loss over 6 months. They randomly assigned overweight or obese men and women with an average body mass index of 31.5 to one of three diet groups: (1) moderate-fat diet (35 to 45 percent fat), (2) low-fat diet (20 to 30 percent fat), or

(3) control diet (35 percent fat). In all three diets, protein constituted 10 to 20 percent. Participants were allowed to eat as much of their assigned diet as they wanted during a 3-week standardization period and 6 months of intervention. After 6 months, the scientists found that none of the diets was superior in preventing weight regain, suggesting that the type of diet you follow is not particularly important for weight maintenance.

In a review of the initial enrollees in the ongoing famous National Weight Control Registry who had lost an average of 66 pounds and maintained the weight loss for an average of 5 years, researchers from the University of Pittsburgh School of Medicine found that the enrollees consumed a low-calorie and low-fat diet after they lost weight. Specifically, women in the registry consumed an average of 1,306 calories per day, with 24.3 percent of those calories from fat, and men consumed an average of 1,685 calories per day, with 23.5 percent of those calories from fat.

Hopefully, you have gotten the message by now that the quantity of calories matters more for weight loss than does the specific combination of macronutrients. However, one clever way to control the quantity of calories is by improving the *quality* of calories. Foods of high nutritional quality, including those that contain protein, make you feel fuller on fewer calories. Indeed, protein makes you feel fuller than does carbohydrate or fat. That is why studies show that high-protein diets are effective for both weight loss and for weight maintenance after weight loss— because of the greater satiety from the protein and resulting reduction in total daily calories. One of these studies comes from the University of Washington School of Medicine, in which researchers placed volunteers on a baseline diet consisting of 35 percent fat, 50 percent carbohydrate, and 15 percent protein for 2 weeks. After blood work and other measurements were taken, the volunteers were placed on a high-protein diet of the same number of calories consisting of 20 percent fat, 50 percent carbohydrate, and 30 percent protein for 2 weeks. After some more measurements, the diet changed again. This time, the macronutrient distribution remained fixed at 20 percent fat, 50 percent carbohydrate, and 30 percent protein for 12 weeks, but the number of calories was not controlled—the volunteers were told to eat as much as they wanted of the supplied diet. The researchers found that the high-protein diet (30 percent of calories) resulted in a clear decrease in hunger and increase in fullness among the volunteers. During the 12 weeks that they were told to eat as much of the high-protein diet as they wanted, they consumed an average of 441 *fewer* calories per day. As a result, they lost an average of nearly 11 pounds, which was fully accounted for by the reduction in caloric intake.

" ONE CLEVER WAY TO CONTROL THE QUANTITY OF CALORIES IS BY IMPROVING THE QUALITY OF CALORIES."

Not only does protein fill you up, it takes a lot of energy to break down dietary protein into its amino acid constituents that are used for metabolism and storage. In simple terms, your body burns more calories to break down and store the protein you eat than it does to break down and store carbohydrate and fat.

Are you confused yet? The truth is that there is no one approach or one diet that works for everyone. This is what all the other books and magazines miss. They cite one study and base a whole program around it. That may work for some people or for a little while, but for safe and sustained weight loss, there are no shortcuts and no magic bullets. Taking the findings of all the weight-loss research together, we see that moderate-carbohydrate and high-protein diets help you lose weight because their higher-quality nutrition fuels your exercise and keeps you fuller. But primarily we see that the exact macronutrient composition isn't really important to losing weight; what's really important is reducing calories.

According to the Food and Nutrition Board of the Institutes of Medicine (IOM), the acceptable macronutrient distribution ranges for active people are 45 to 65 percent carbohydrate, 10 to 35 percent protein, and 20 to 35 percent fat. If you stick to 1,500 calories per day, that means you could eat 675 to 975 grams of carbohydrate, 150 to 525 grams of protein, and 300 to 525 grams of fat per day. You'll notice there's quite a bit of variation in these numbers. Variety is the spice of nutrition, after all. The *Run Your Fat Off* nutrition menu includes slightly less carbohydrate, since a number of studies support the consumption of a lower percentage of carbohydrate to lose weight.

It's not critical to balance the macronutrients to the exact percentage or number of grams throughout the day. And not all meals have to be, or even should be, of the same distribution. As long as you eat enough to meet your body's needs and to support your running habit, you'll be fine. In fact, you'll be better than fine—you'll be a supercharged engine ready to run, look, and feel the best you ever have.

NUTRIENT TIMING

It's obvious that how much you eat has a significant impact on your ability to lose weight. *When* you eat, and specifically when you eat different macronutrients, can also impact your ability to lose weight, although the effects are more subtle.

Within 30 to 60 minutes of consuming carbohydrate, insulin increases up to eight-fold in response to the increased glucose in your blood. Since insulin governs glucose metabolism, the best time to consume carbohydrate and thus increase insulin is either first thing in the morning when you need carbohydrate for fuel or immediately after running when you need to replenish the carbohydrate that was used.

When it comes to weight loss, it turns out that your mother was right after all—breakfast really is the most important meal of the day. Because blood glucose is lower in the morning from your overnight fast, the carbohydrate you eat at breakfast will be used to replenish your blood glucose and muscle glycogen rather than be stored as fat. Also, skipping breakfast makes you hungry and therefore more likely to eat a lot more later in the day to compensate. Research has shown that a high-caloric intake during breakfast results in greater weight loss than a high-caloric intake during dinner. Scientists at Tel Aviv University placed 93 overweight and obese women on two diets containing identical macronutrient content and composition equaling 1,400 calories for 12 weeks. The only difference was that one diet emphasized a big breakfast (50 percent of daily calories) and a small dinner (14 percent of daily calories) and the other diet emphasized a big dinner and a small breakfast by reversing the percentages. After 12 weeks, the women on the high-calorie breakfast lost nearly two and a half times more weight than those on the high-calorie dinner (19 vs. 8 pounds, respectively). Waist circumference and BMI also decreased more with the high-calorie breakfast than with the high-calorie dinner.

But breakfast is not the only meal that matters. Scientists at the University of Murcia in Spain studied the effects of lunchtime on weight loss in 420 individuals over 20 weeks. In this Mediterranean population, lunch was the main meal of the day, with 40 percent of daily calories consumed. Among the participants in the study, 51 percent were classified as early eaters (lunchtime before 3 p.m.) and 49 percent were classified as late eaters (lunchtime after 3 p.m.). The scientists found that, starting after the

WATER

Despite what you see when you look in the mirror, water, not muscle or fat, is the major component of your body, making up about 60 percent of your body weight. Water is vital for most chemical reactions that occur inside your cells, including the production of energy (ATP) for muscle contraction. Drinking water throughout the day is not only important for the chemistry of your cells, it also keeps your stomach full so you aren't tempted to eat more.

Most people consume a lot of unnecessary calories from beverages, which can easily thwart your weight-loss plans. Indeed, some people actually drink more calories than they eat. Sodas, smoothies, coffee drinks, and fruit juice can contribute significantly to total calories and become a big obstacle to weight loss. To eliminate unnecessary calories, water should be the predominant, if not the only, thing you drink. A single 12-ounce can of Coca-Cola is 140 calories (which would take almost 1.5 miles of running to burn), with zero of those calories being nutritious. Even diet soda still contains artificial sweeteners and acts like sugar in raising insulin level and promoting weight gain. Replacing soda with water is perhaps the easiest way to consume fewer calories and keep your stomach full at the same time.

When you lose water through dieting, sweating, or even through breathing (yes, breathing), your body temperature increases when you run. In an attempt to prevent body temperature from rising to dangerous levels, your central nervous system orchestrates a complex response in which blood vessels supplying your muscles and other organs constrict while blood vessels supplying your skin dilate. This causes blood to be diverted from your muscles and other organs toward your skin in order to increase cooling through the convection of air over your skin's surface. With less blood (and thus oxygen) flow to your muscles, your pace slows down.

If you don't consume enough water to replace what you've lost, your blood volume also decreases and becomes thicker, which reduces your heart's stroke volume, cardiac output, and, ultimately, oxygen delivery. Your running performance starts to decline with only a 2 to 3 percent loss of body weight due to fluid loss.

To rehydrate after a long run (of an hour or more), drink fluids that contain sodium, which stimulates your kidneys to retain water. If your run is less than an hour, plain water in combination with a balanced diet is just as effective. Since most drinks contain excess calories that you don't need, plain water is best. A good indicator of your hydration level is the color of your urine, with a light color like lemonade indicating that you're adequately hydrated. By contrast, if your urine looks like apple juice, keep drinking. The IOM recommends that men drink at least 12.5 cups (0.8 gallon) per day and women drink at least 9 cups (0.6 gallon) per day. That's a lot of water!

fifth week, early-lunch eaters lost more weight more quickly than did late-lunch eaters. Early-lunch eaters also consumed a greater percentage of their daily calories at breakfast and skipped breakfast less often than late-lunch eaters did. The effect of lunchtime on weight loss was independent of other factors affecting weight loss, including caloric intake, macronutrient composition, estimated energy expenditure, appetite hormones, and sleep duration, as all of these factors were similar between the early- and late-lunch eaters. Although it is not currently known why the timing of meals affects weight loss, meal timing may affect the circadian rhythm control of hormones that regulate hunger.

Timing your meals to your runs also influences whether your calories are used to satisfy metabolic demands or stored as body fat. Apart from breakfast and lunch, most of your carbohydrate should come immediately after your runs. Muscles are picky when it comes to the time for synthesizing and storing glycogen, because they are extremely sensitive to the effects of insulin (aerobic exercise like running on a regular basis increases the muscles' sensitivity to insulin), which increases immediately after consuming carbohydrate. Muscles want carbohydrate within 45 minutes after your workouts.

If you run *before* breakfast, when blood glucose is already low from your overnight fast, the carbohydrate you eat at breakfast is more likely to be stored as glycogen than as fat because of the metabolic demand you have created. (You will still have enough energy to run before breakfast.) Running before breakfast (i.e., fasted runs) can also help you reduce the total number of calories you consume during the day, especially if you run later in the morning, since you'll have fewer hours in the day to eat.

Protein is another important nutrient to consume after you run, and especially when you are trying to build muscle. As with carbohydrate, when you consume protein immediately after your workouts, especially resistance workouts, the amino acids from that protein will be used to build muscle rather than be stored as fat.

◆ ◆ ◆ ◆ ◆

THE MOTIVATION TO LOSE WEIGHT can come from anywhere. Sometimes it comes from an unexpected place. Professor Mark Haub's motivation came from his classroom. "I needed a reason to start to lose weight," he says. "The class project was that spark to start." And so 40-year-old Mark Haub became the lone subject in his own Energy Balance class experiment and went on what became known in the media as the Twinkie diet. For 10 weeks, instead of eating breakfast, lunch, and dinner, he ate a Twinkie every 3 hours. He also munched on other convenience store snacks—Doritos chips, sugary cereals, and Oreos—so he wouldn't get bored with eating just Twinkies. "The obesogenic foods stated in the USDA guidelines were the basis for the foods that were chosen for our project," he says. So he wouldn't completely sacrifice his health, he took a multivitamin and drank a protein shake daily and ate some vegetables at dinner, typically a can of green beans or a few celery stalks. He limited himself to less than 1,800 calories per day, averaging about 1,650 calories per day. Two-thirds of those calories came from the saturated fat of junk food. He also continued his modest level of exercise that he did before beginning the experiment.

Mark's Twinkie diet, which was really only meant to be a small class project, got a fair amount of press. He was a guest on *The Doctors* and *Good Morning America*. He lost 27 pounds in 10 weeks, his body fat dropped from 33.4 percent to 24.9 percent, and his BMI dropped from 28.8 to 24.9. And traditional markers of his health improved—his "bad" LDL cholesterol dropped by 20 percent, his "good" HDL cholesterol increased by 20 percent, and his triglycerides, which are a measure of fat in the bloodstream, dropped by 39 percent. Despite the "unhealthy" food he ate, the weight loss he experienced caused him to become "healthier," at least as defined by his percent body fat, BMI, and blood lipid profile. Weight loss by itself makes you healthier by improving your blood lipid profile and decreasing cardiovascular risk factors. Before his Twinkie diet, Mark tried to eat a "healthy" diet that included whole grains, fiber, berries, bananas, and vegetables, with only the occasional treats like pizza. But he didn't lose weight. "There seems to be a disconnect between eating healthy and being healthy," he says. "It may not be the same. I was eating healthier, but I wasn't healthy. I was eating too much."

Despite the public's perception of junk food and what we're told we shouldn't eat, Mark says the process of losing weight on the Twinkie diet was relatively easy, although it wasn't without some challenges. "I learned how easy anorexic-type thoughts—'If I don't eat this snack or dinner, I can weigh even less tomorrow'—can occur," he admits. "Portion size was my issue."

Although I don't recommend you add Twinkies and Ding Dongs to the *Run Your Fat Off* meal plan after every meal, Mark's experiment underscores the point that the number of calories you consume relative to how many you expend—more than any other issue—is what influences your body weight. We return to Albert Einstein and his famous equation: $E = mc^2$. If you consume more energy (calories) than what you expend through exercise and other physical activity, you will store that energy on your body and you will gain mass; if you expend more energy than what you consume, you will lose mass. Look at the equation: If energy increases, mass increases by the same amount because energy and mass are proportional; if energy decreases, mass decreases by the same amount because energy and mass are proportional. The truth is, if you commit to the physical work, all of the food you eat (as long as you don't overeat relative to your caloric expenditure), no matter what that food is, will be used as fuel. None of it will collect on your butt.

You can eat too much "bad" food and you can eat too much "good" food. However, it's important to eat nutritious foods that satiate you so you limit how hungry you feel throughout the day. When you eat a lot of junk food, it's easy to overeat because the junk food is not satiating. Try eating a single chocolate chip cookie versus a kale salad. They may be the same number of calories, but the kale salad will be filling, while the hunger you'll experience after eating the single chocolate chip cookie will have you reaching for another one. That's why it was hard for Mark to eat fewer calories on the Twinkie diet.

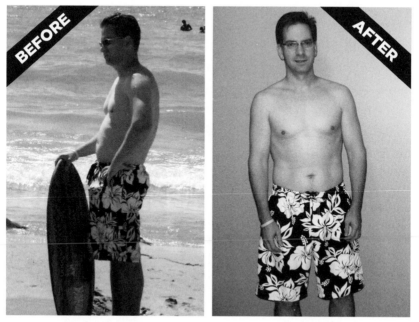

**Dr. Mark Haub
at 201 pounds.**

**Haub now,
at 174 pounds.**

That the number of calories matter was not the only thing Mark learned from his class project. He also gained an interesting perspective on diets in general. "I discovered how vitriolic people can be when they take a stance, whether it's a low-carb or Paleo diet or something else. It's like politics or religion. Those discussions can get heated: 'I'm right. You're wrong.' We have this mantra in our society: 'Don't eat this, don't eat that.' While no one *needs* to eat a cookie, it's okay for someone to eat a cookie twice a week." Same goes for Twinkies. It's okay to have unhealthy snacks from time to time, as long as those junk food items don't displace other healthy foods in your diet and as long as you still meet your daily needs for all other nutrients.

The truth is that there is no "best" diet. All diets—even the Twinkie diet—can work if they provide a caloric deficit and you stick with them. "From a food and fitness perspective, people need to figure out what their bodies need," Mark says.

Mark no longer follows the Twinkie diet, having gone back to eating more "healthy" foods after completing the class project. "Now I have to be more mindful about what I eat," he says, lest he gain the weight back. "I have decreased my meal size since the experiment, which is a positive outcome for me."

Mark doesn't run much, if at all, these days, having badly hurt his knee playing baseball while coaching his kids. But as a former collegiate runner, he recognizes the effectiveness of running for weight loss. "When I was at my lowest level of body fat, I was running 85 miles per week," he says. "When I was running a lot, it was a struggle to keep weight *on*."

CHAPTER 6

The *Run Your Fat Off* Nutrition Menus

**"ONE NIGHT, AS I WAS WALKING ON IT,
I THOUGHT, 'I WONDER IF I COULD RUN ON THIS THING?'"**

JEN HUDSON MOSHER grew up a chubby child in a small town in northern New York. There was never a time when she was in shape. During a routine physical exam her senior year of high school as she prepared to go to college, she discovered that she weighed 202 pounds. "For most anyone, that's fat," she says, "but at my height of 5-foot-1, I was obese."

Over the next 4 years, she lived the typical college lifestyle of drinking lots of soda and eating unhealthy foods, and she continued to gain weight. She tried a couple of times, she says, to get into healthy living—eating better and visiting the gym on campus—but those efforts were short-lived. During her freshman year, her father died of a heart attack. He was only 42 years old. "I was worried that was destined to be my fate as well," she says.

After graduating from college, she moved back home, first with her mother, then with her boyfriend, who is now her husband. "I ate fast food at least 5 days a week. And I got virtually no exercise," she says. "By the time my boyfriend and I moved in together, I couldn't shop in regular stores; as a size 34, they didn't have clothes large enough to fit me. I was working as a professional and had to buy clothes for fat women online without trying anything on."

Jen knew that she was morbidly obese, but she rationalized that her weight issue wasn't that bad. "I would take frequent 2-mile walks with our dogs and had no major health issues, so I was good," she says. "I would tell myself that I was just destined to be heavy and nothing could change that."

In her early thirties, Jen started to experience symptoms related to being obese. She was diagnosed with severe sleep apnea, a disorder common in overweight people in which breathing is briefly and repeatedly interrupted during sleep. And her knees ached all the time. "Walking up a flight of stairs was a monumental task," she says.

In February 2010, at age 37, she reached her heaviest weight. "I can remember walking into the doctor's office and getting on the scale; it read 344 pounds. I was larger than most NFL linebackers!" Something had to change.

◆ ◆ ◆ ◆ ◆

YOU WON'T FIND A MAGIC PILL or secret sauce or a diet named after our ancestors in the *Run Your Fat Off* diet, but you will find a plan that works. There's no restricting what you eat, only how much of it you eat and when you eat it. People trying to lose weight are often hard on themselves about what and how much they eat. Don't be. You're human, after all. Bad, high-caloric food tastes good, and it's not always easy to run when life gets in the way. Just always keep your goals at the forefront of your mind and let those goals be your guide to keep you on the right path.

Eat until you're satisfied, not stuffed. If you feel bloated after eating, you ate too much. Eat slower so that you have a better sense of when you become satisfied. If you eat too fast, you'll have eaten all of the calories before realizing that you're satisfied.

The *Run Your Fat Off* diet is about weight loss, health, and providing you with the right fuels for running, which helps you avoid injuries and illness, maximizes your running performance, and assists in recovery from your workouts. Only in America is the philosophy to eat first and then work. We say things like, "I have to go to the gym tomorrow to work off this meal." Imagine if we applied the same reasoning to our cars. We don't fill up our cars with gasoline and then say, "I have to drive a lot tomorrow to burn off all this gasoline." We drive a car and then put gasoline in it so we can drive it again tomorrow. We see gasoline as fuel for driving a car. So why don't we see food as fuel to drive our bodies? Runners do. I have never viewed running as a way to burn off the big meal I just ate. I run and then I eat to refuel so I can feel good on my run tomorrow. When physical work comes before food rather than the other way around, your health and your life will change for the better. View the food you consume as your nutrition plan to fuel and recover from your running and you'll never have to go on a diet again.

One of the reasons it's hard to stick to most diets is because of their rigidity. Nearly all diets restrict *something* and many diets restrict *a lot of things*. When you run a lot, the extra calories you burn give you more flexibility. You can eat a few chocolate chip cookies and it won't destroy your weight-loss goals. If you don't run, your diet becomes everything; no chocolate chip cookies allowed.

That being said, as we've discussed, it's faster and easier to affect your waistline initally by eating less than by running. To get a jump start on losing weight, try cutting about 300 to 500 calories out of your day. Once you start running or focus on running more, you can expect to be hungry, which will make eating fewer calories difficult. So get used to eating fewer calories for a few weeks first. Then, when you start your running plan or increase how much you run, you'll be able to achieve a bigger calorie deficit more easily.

I would love to include a nutrition menu for eating 3 days, 4 days, and 5 days per week. Unfortunately, that wouldn't fly since people need to eat every day. Given that you do need to eat every day, you need to control *how much* you eat every day yet limit hunger so you are not tempted or compelled to eat more. The specific macronutrients and micronutrients, the timing of when you eat, and the amount you drink all influence your hunger. To limit hunger while cutting calories, the *Run Your Fat Off* diet includes nutrient-dense foods that make you feel full.

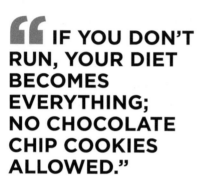

IF YOU DON'T RUN, YOUR DIET BECOMES EVERYTHING; NO CHOCOLATE CHIP COOKIES ALLOWED."

All meals on the menu have been developed with nutrient analysis software to meet specific nutrient configurations of 35 to 45 percent carbohydrate (a little lower than the Institutes of Medicine ranges noted in Chapter 5, as studies support a lower percentage of carbohydrate to lose weight), 20 to 35 percent protein, and 20 to 35 percent fat, and highlights other nutrients, including fiber, to make sure you get exactly what you need. Fiber helps you feel full so you eat less, which contributes to your weight-loss goal. It also decreases the risk for chronic diseases, including diabetes, cardiovascular disease, and some cancers.

Rather than giving you a meal plan that makes you stick to a specific daily diet, our menu is flexible and provides the percentages of carbohydrate, protein, and fat for every meal option. With five options each for breakfast, lunch, dinner, and snacks, the *Run Your Fat Off* menu gives you 625 total combinations so you'll never get bored. Select one option from each meal and snack per day to develop your own unique combination of meals and snacks. You can mix and match meals between categories (e.g., swap a lunch for a dinner) as long as you maintain the overall calorie count. Eat one of your meals within an hour after your run, especially if you do double runs or do a second nonrunning workout on the same day.

You can also manipulate your carbohydrate composition in concert with your runs. For example, on days that you run longer or faster, choose a breakfast that is a little higher in carbs so that you have enough energy to get through the workout feeling good. On days that you have a shorter or less intense run, choose one of the lower-carbohydrate breakfasts, regardless of the time of day you run.

You may be happy to see some desserts in the *Run Your Fat Off* diet. While it's important to indulge in desserts once in a while because you shouldn't go through life denying yourself the foods (and the experiences of those foods) that taste good, don't have one after every meal or even every day. That will only thwart your weight-loss plan. Limit the number of desserts you eat each week to one or two.

All of the recipes in this chapter make one serving. If you would like to make more to have leftovers later in the week, simply double or triple the quantities.

THE
RUN YOUR FAT OFF
MENUS

◆ ◆ ◆

VEGETARIAN AND VEGAN SUBSTITUTES

If you are vegan or vegetarian, use the following chart to make appropriate substitutes for the meat and/or dairy products in the following meals and recipes. Note that this will change the nutrition information for each meal slightly, but all meals will remain healthy, menu-compliant choices.

FOR	SUBSTITUTE
egg whites and turkey bacon	veggie sausage patty or veggie bacon
cow milk yogurt	soy-, almond-, or coconut-cultured milks
scrambled egg and egg white dishes	vegan egg
animal protein ounce-for-ounce substitution (e.g., shrimp, fish, beef, etc.)	plant protein (e.g., tempeh, seitan, tofu, or legumes)

Breakfast

◆

(250 to 300 calories)
CHOOSE 1 BREAKFAST EACH DAY

Veggie and Cheese Egg White Frittata

*A five egg white, open-faced omelet filled
with steamed broccoli and topped with gooey melted
Swiss cheese. Served with a tender baked apple*

299 calories: 37% carbohydrate, 37% protein, 26% fat, 7g fiber

High in riboflavin (vitamin B_2), an important vitamin
for energy production

◆

Salsa Egg Scramble Roll-Up

*Warm rolled corn tortilla stuffed with scrambled eggs
and flavorful salsa. Served with ½ cup grapes*

289 calories: 36% carbohydrate, 20% protein, 44% fat, 2g fiber

About half of the daily requirement for phosphorus,
a mineral important for muscle contraction

◆

Nutty Cinnamon Oatmeal

*Wholesome nutty and aromatic oatmeal
with cinnamon and chopped walnuts. Served
with hard-boiled egg whites and turkey bacon*

285 calories: 37% carbohydrate, 32% protein, 31% fat, 5g fiber

Very high in iron, an important mineral for oxygenating blood

Apple and Peanut Butter Toast

Heart-healthy peanut butter on toasted whole-grain goodness, topped with crispy tart apple. Served with turkey bacon

268 calories: 42% carbohydrate, 21% protein, 37% fat, 5g fiber

More than half of the daily requirement for manganese, important for bone production and blood sugar control

Strawberry Walnut Yogurt Parfait

A layered treat of creamy berry and Greek yogurts, heart-healthy walnuts, and juicy strawberries

300 calories: 47% carbohydrate, 22% protein, 31% fat, 8g fiber

Loaded with vitamin C, an important antioxidant for immune function

Lunch

◆

(350 to 400 calories)
CHOOSE 1 LUNCH EACH DAY

Tuna Melt

A mouthwatering trio of tuna, melted cheddar cheese,
and whole-wheat English muffin broiled to perfection.
Served with 1 cup of strawberries

400 calories: 42% carbohydrate, 37% protein, 21% fat, 5g fiber

Contains heart-healthy omega-3 fatty acids
important for fighting inflammation

◆

Classic Soup and Half Sandwich

Delicious cup of heart-healthy lentil soup and turkey
half sandwich loaded with crunchy veggies and tangy tomato

359 calories: 50% carbohydrate, 34% protein, 16% fat, 5g fiber

A hefty dose of vitamin B_{12}, a major player
in metabolism and nervous system function

◆

Quick Chicken Pizza

A delicioso version of an Italian classic, with grilled chicken,
tangy tomato sauce, and gooey cheese

356 calories: 39% carbohydrate, 36% protein, 25% fat, 2g fiber

Almost 100 percent of the daily requirement for niacin,
a vitamin that raises "good" HDL cholesterol

◆

Turkey and Cheese Roll-Up

*A mini wrap of smoked turkey rolled around a
cheddar cheese chunk. Served with a side of raisins*

388 calories: 43% carbohydrate, 35% protein, 22% fat, 2g fiber

A hefty dose of vitamin B_{12}, a major player
in metabolism and nervous system function

◆

Chef Salad

*A giant bowl of tossed lettuce, tomato, savory turkey strips,
and wholesome hard-boiled egg, drizzled with low-fat dressing*

362 calories: 42% carbohydrate, 37% protein, 21% fat, 6g fiber

With 6g of fiber, this salad will keep you full for hours

Dinner

◆

(400 to 500 calories)
CHOOSE 1 DINNER EACH DAY

Teriyaki-Glazed Salmon

*Perfectly broiled salmon in teriyaki sauce served
with brown rice and steamed broccoli with lemon*

426 calories: 42% carbohydrate, 33% protein, 25% fat, 3g fiber

A hefty dose of vitamin B_{12}, a major player in metabolism and nervous
system function, and high in anti-inflammatory omega-3 fatty acids

◆

Garlic Shrimp Linguini

*Grilled shrimp and marinated artichokes served over a bed
of linguini and drizzled with olive oil and Parmesan cheese*

481 calories: 40% carbohydrate, 27% protein, 33% fat, 9g fiber

Very high in selenium, a potent antioxidant
to protect cells from damage

◆

Turkey Burger 'n' Fries

*A sizzling hot turkey burger stuffed with
sautéed onions and served with baked fries*

472 calories: 41% carbohydrate, 25% protein, 34% fat, 5g fiber

More than half the daily requirement for vitamin B_6,
which is involved in more than 100 metabolic reactions

Filet Mignon with Arugula Salad

*A tender steak filet cooked to juicy perfection
served with a peppery arugula, pear,
and goat cheese salad sprinkled with raisins*

499 calories: 40% carbohydrate, 25% protein, 35% fat, 7g fiber

High in vitamin B_{12}, a major player in metabolism
and nervous system function

Garden Omelet

*A veggie medley of broccoli, mushrooms, and tomatoes
with cheddar cheese wrapped inside a fluffy two-egg omelet
served with a slice of whole-wheat toast and an orange*

408 calories: 38% carbohydrate, 25% protein, 37% fat, 8g fiber

Almost double the daily requirement for vitamin C,
an important antioxidant for immune function

Snacks

◆

(150 to 250 calories)

CHOOSE 1 TO 2 SNACKS EACH DAY

PB and Celery
(vegan)

Large, crisp celery stalk filled with
2 tablespoons all-natural peanut butter

194 calories: 16% carbohydrate, 15% protein, 69% fat, 3g fiber

◆

Trail Mix
(vegan)

Tasty blend of almonds, walnuts, raisins, and apricots

174 calories: 46% carbohydrate, 8% protein, 46% fat, 3g fiber

◆

Egg Salad Rice Cake

Creamy hard-boiled egg salad on a crunchy rice cake

157 calories: 24% carbohydrate, 19% protein, 57% fat, <1g fiber

◆

Hummus and Carrots
(vegan)

Baby carrots dipped in 5 ounces savory hummus

152 calories: 53% carbohydrate, 10% protein, 37% fat, 2g fiber

◆

Salsa-Filled Avocado
(vegan)

Avocado stuffed with tangy salsa

153 calories: 37% carbohydrate, 9% protein, 54% fat, 7g fiber

Dessert

◆

(100 to 225 calories)

CHOOSE 1 TO 2 DESSERTS EACH WEEK

Vanilla Bean Fruit Salad

*A sumptuous combo of your favorite seasonal fruit
with vanilla bean whipped topping*

164 calories: 88% carbohydrate, 7% protein, 5% fat, 2g fiber

◆

Creamy Chocolate Pudding

Creamy chocolate pudding with cocoa-infused whipped topping

206 calories: 72% carbohydrate, 16% protein, 12% fat, 1g fiber (with sugar)
142 calories: 60% carbohydrate, 23% protein, 17% fat, 1g fiber
(with a non-nutritive sugar substitute, such as Splenda, Equal, or Stevia)

◆

Ginger-Laced Baked Apple

*Bubbling cinnamon-sugar baked apple
with spicy ginger whipped topping*

142 calories: 91% carbohydrate, 4% protein, 5% fat, 4g fiber

◆

Peanut Butter Oat No-Bake Cookies

*Rolled peanut butter oats with spiced brown sugar
notes and chock-full of raisins*

222 calories: 64% carbohydrate, 10% protein, 26% fat, 3g fiber

Beverages

◆

Water

◆

Flavored Water

*(with lemon, lime, or cucumber, or commercially available waters
with flavors, such as lemon-flavored Perrier,
with no added sugar or calories)*

◆

Black Coffee

◆

Tea

◆

Seltzer, Club Soda,
or Other Carbonated Water

◆

Spritzer

8 ounces seltzer mixed with 3 tablespoons juice

◆

Diet Soda

Artificial (noncaloric) sweeteners can be used for taste

THE
RUN YOUR FAT OFF
RECIPES

◆ ◆ ◆

Breakfast Recipes

Veggie and Cheese Egg White Frittata

5 egg whites
½ cup chopped broccoli, steamed
1 oz. grated Swiss cheese

Preheat broiler on high. Spray nonstick 8-inch or medium skillet with nonstick spray. Over low heat, add egg whites to skillet and cook until they start to bubble (about 3 to 5 minutes). Sprinkle broccoli and Swiss cheese over entire surface. Place skillet under broiler for 1 to 2 minutes, watching that frittata doesn't burn. When egg white is cooked through, remove from oven and slide off skillet. Serve with a baked apple.

Baked Apple

1 apple
1 tbsp. cinnamon
1 packet artificial sweetener (optional)
½ cup water

Preheat oven to 375°F. Keeping apple whole, remove as much of the core as possible from the top with a sharp paring knife, and follow with a small spoon to remove seeds. Fill the well with cinnamon and (if desired) one packet of artificial sweetener. Pour water in glass baking pan of any size and place apple in pan so apple sits in one-eighth inch of water. Bake for 30 to 45 minutes until apple is cooked through and tender.

Note: Can be refrigerated and reheated at later time.

Salsa Egg Scramble Roll-Up

1 egg
1 oz. (¼ cup) shredded Swiss cheese
1 corn 8-inch tortilla, warmed in oven
3 tbsp. salsa
½ cup grapes

Spray skillet (any size) with nonstick spray. Scramble egg in skillet and add cheese. Spread scrambled egg and cheese over tortilla and cover with salsa. Roll up and enjoy with a side of grapes.

Nutty Cinnamon Oatmeal

2 packets instant or ½ cup steel-cut oatmeal
Water per oatmeal directions
½ tsp. cinnamon
⅛ cup chopped walnuts
2 hard-boiled egg whites
4 slices turkey bacon

Prepare oatmeal (instant or long cooking) as directed, adding cinnamon toward end of cooking time. Spoon into bowl. Add chopped walnuts. Serve with egg whites and turkey bacon.

Apple and Peanut Butter Toast

1 slice whole-wheat bread
1 tbsp. natural peanut butter
1 apple, sliced
1 slice turkey bacon

Toast bread to desired preference. Spread peanut butter on toast. Top with apple slices and serve with turkey bacon.

Strawberry Walnut Yogurt Parfait

$\frac{1}{2}$ cup low-fat berry yogurt
$\frac{1}{2}$ cup nonfat Greek vanilla or plain yogurt
1 cup fresh (or frozen) sliced strawberries
$\frac{1}{8}$ cup chopped walnuts

In a clear parfait glass or cup, layer a few tablespoons each of berry yogurt, Greek yogurt, sliced strawberries, and a sprinkle of walnuts.

Lunch Recipes

Tuna Melt

½ (5-oz.) can water-packed tuna (preferably light)
1 tbsp. low-fat mayonnaise
1 tsp. mustard (any type)
Salt, pepper, & herb seasonings
½ whole-wheat English muffin
1 (1-oz.) slice cheddar cheese

Preheat broiler to high. Mix tuna, mayonnaise, and mustard in small bowl. Add salt, pepper, and other spices to taste. Set aside. Split English muffin and save half for later use. Spread tuna mixture on half. Top with cheddar cheese. Place under broiler until cheese melts (1 to 3 minutes).

Classic Soup and Half Sandwich

1 cup lentil soup (any heart-healthy commercial brand)
1 tsp. mustard (Dijon or yellow)
1 slice whole-wheat bread, cut in half
3 oz. turkey breast, sliced
2 leaves Bibb or romaine lettuce
2 slices ripe tomato
4 slices cucumber, with peel

Heat soup in small saucepan over medium heat until almost boiling. Spread mustard evenly on both half slices of bread. Place turkey, lettuce, tomato, and cucumber slices on top of one-half slice of bread and top with second half slice of bread.

Quick Chicken Pizza

1 large pita bread, halved lengthwise
1/2 cup tomato sauce
2 oz. grilled or roasted chicken, diced
1/2 cup shredded low-fat mozzarella cheese
Garlic powder, oregano, pepper flakes, & other desired spices

Place half pita bread "inside up" on cookie sheet. Spread with tomato sauce, add chicken, and sprinkle with mozzarella and herbs of choice. Place in broiler on high until cheese melts and sauce bubbles (about 2 to 3 minutes).

Turkey and Cheese Roll-Up

1 slice smoked turkey lunchmeat
1 oz. aged cheddar cheese
1 small box (1 oz.) raisins

Wrap turkey slice twice around cheese. Serve with raisins.

Chef Salad

3 cups torn lettuce
1 medium tomato, diced
2 oz. turkey (or ham) lunchmeat
1 hard-boiled egg, diced
2 tbsp. low-calorie salad dressing
8 whole wheat crackers

Mix lettuce, tomatoes, turkey (or ham), egg, and salad dressing in large bowl. Serve with crackers.

Dinner Recipes

Teriyaki-Glazed Salmon

1 (4-oz.) salmon fillet

2 tbsp. teriyaki sauce

½ cup ready-to-eat or already-cooked brown rice

1 cup broccoli florets, steamed

1 lemon wedge

Place salmon fillet in plastic zip-lock bag with teriyaki sauce and let marinate in refrigerator for 4 to 8 hours. When ready to cook, remove salmon from bag and place on small baking dish sprayed with nonstick spray. Place in broiler on high for 6 to 10 minutes until salmon flakes and appears cooked through. Serve with brown rice and steamed broccoli with a squeeze of lemon.

Garlic Shrimp Linguini

1 tbsp. olive oil

1 clove garlic, diced

3 oz. (about 12) peeled medium shrimp

½ jar marinated artichoke hearts, diced

4 oz. (about 1 ½ cups) cooked linguini

1 tbsp. Parmesan cheese

In 8-inch or medium skillet, heat olive oil on low and sauté garlic until golden. Add shrimp and cook until pink, about 5 to 7 minutes. Add diced artichoke hearts and cook on low for 3 minutes. Place linguini in bowl and toss with shrimp and artichoke mixture. Sprinkle Parmesan on top and serve.

Turkey Burger 'n' Fries

1 small onion, sliced in thin rounds
3 oz. ground turkey
1 small Idaho potato, sliced in shoestrings
1 ½ tsp. olive oil
Salt and pepper to taste

To make the burger: Spray 8-inch or medium skillet with nonstick spray and sauté onions until translucent. Make ball out of ground turkey and press a well into ball with thumb. Fill well with sautéed onions, and flatten slightly into a thick patty. Cook patty over low heat in a nonstick skillet for 5 minutes each side.

To make the fries: Slice potato into shoestrings and toss in a bowl with olive oil (salt and pepper if desired). Spread potatoes on baking sheet and bake at 375°F for 20 minutes, tossing every 5 minutes to cook on all sides.

Filet Mignon with Arugula Salad

3 oz. filet mignon
2 cups arugula
1 oz. goat cheese, torn into loose pieces
1 Bartlett pear, cored and thinly sliced
1 tbsp. raisins
1 tbsp. nonfat salad dressing

Spray 8-inch or medium skillet with nonstick spray and sauté filet mignon, turning frequently so that it cooks through (10 to 20 minutes, depending on thickness and desired degree of doneness). Place arugula in bowl with torn goat cheese, sliced pear, and raisins. Toss with low-fat dressing of choice.

Garden Omelet

2 eggs
1 ½ cups combined broccoli florets, sliced mushrooms, and diced tomato
1 oz. shredded cheddar cheese
1 slice whole-wheat toast
1 orange

Scramble eggs in small bowl. Spray 8-inch or medium skillet with nonstick spray and sauté vegetables until soft. Set aside. Pour eggs into skillet and let cook until bottom begins to bubble. Pour cooked vegetables and cheese over top and place under broiler on high for 1 to 2 minutes to cook through. Fold omelet in half. Serve with whole-wheat toast and orange.

Snack Recipes

Trail Mix

5 almonds
5 walnut halves
1 tbsp. raisins
6 dried apricot halves

In small serving bowl, mix almonds, walnut halves, raisins, and dried apricot halves.

Egg Salad Rice Cake

1 hard-boiled egg, diced
2 tbsp. reduced-fat mayonnaise
1 tsp. mustard
1 rice cake

Mix diced egg with mayonnaise and mustard. Scoop mixture onto rice cake.

Salsa-Filled Avocado

1 avocado
½ cup salsa (store-bought)

Slice avocado in half and remove pit. Fill each half of avocado with salsa.

Dessert Recipes

Vanilla Bean Fruit Salad

1 1/2 cups diced seasonal fruit
1/4 cup low-fat vanilla whipped topping
Lime juice

Toss diced fruit in medium bowl with a squirt of lime juice and refrigerate. Top with vanilla whipped cream (see recipe on page 172). Can be enjoyed for 2 to 3 days.

Creamy Chocolate Pudding

2 cups 1% milk or canned coconut milk
1/8 tsp. salt
1/4 cup Dutch cocoa powder
1 packet stevia or 1/4 cup sugar
1/2 cup milk
3 tbsp. cornstarch
3/4 tsp. pure vanilla extract

Heat the 2 cups milk in medium saucepan with the salt, cocoa powder, and sweetener. Meanwhile, whisk the 1/2 cup milk and cornstarch in small bowl until dissolved. Add the cornstarch mixture and vanilla to the warm milk and bring to a boil. Once boiling, stir constantly for 2 minutes. Lower to a simmer for an additional minute. Remove from heat and refrigerate overnight to thicken.

Ginger-Laced Baked Apple

1 Honeycrisp, Granny Smith, or Macintosh apple
¼ cup low-fat ginger whipped topping (see below)

Follow baked apple directions from breakfast recipe on page 162. Apple can be cooked alone or in a batch of up to 3 and kept refrigerated for 2 to 3 days. Warm apple in oven before eating. Top with ginger whipped topping.

Whipped Topping (vanilla or ginger)

1 tsp. unflavored gelatin
2 tsp. water
¼ cup nonfat milk powder
½ cup nonfat milk
1 tbsp. sugar
Flavoring: ½ tsp. vanilla extract or ⅛ tsp. powdered ginger or 1 tbsp. cocoa powder

In small bowl, soften gelatin in water for 5 minutes. In medium saucepan, stir milk powder into milk. Heat to simmering. Add softened gelatin and stir until gelatin dissolves. Add sugar and flavoring of choice. Chill until mixture begins to thicken. Beat with electric mixer or rotary beater until very thick and light. Makes 2 cups. May be stored in refrigerator for use within several days or frozen for longer storage.

Note: Add vanilla for Vanilla Bean Fruit Salad and powdered ginger for Ginger-Laced Baked Apple.

Peanut Butter Oat No-Bake Cookies

1/3 cup brown sugar
2 tsp. unsweetened cocoa
2 tbsp. nonfat milk
2 tbsp. all-natural peanut butter
1/4 tsp. vanilla extract
1/2 cup quick-cooking rolled oats
1/4 cup (1 oz.) raisins

Stir together sugar, cocoa, and milk in 4-cup glass measure or medium microwave-safe bowl. Microwave on high for 1 minute or until boiling, stirring once. Stir in peanut butter, vanilla, oats, and raisins until combined. Drop spoonfuls onto waxed paper–lined plate to make 6 cookies. Place in freezer for 10 minutes before serving. Makes 3 servings.

◆ ◆ ◆ ◆ ◆

Jen Hudson Mosher has been sober from soda for 7 years. "I went from drinking two to three Mountain Dews per day to two to three per week and then to none," she says. "I last drank soda in May 2010." She also began walking on a regular basis, stopped eating fast food, and said no to cake at office parties. "I started reading about healthy foods and incorporating them into my life."

By fall of that year, she had lost about 50 pounds. The weather was getting cold, so she bought a treadmill to use at home. "One night, as I was walking on it, I thought, 'I wonder if I could run on this thing?' I had *never* run in my life. I cranked the treadmill up to 4.5 miles per hour and ran for 30 seconds. I weighed 289 pounds at the time."

From there, Jen started to incorporate running into her nightly walks. "I ran slowly and it hurt," she says. "I can remember the first time I ran 2 minutes straight; I thought I was going to die. I hated it . . . and loved it at the same time."

Jen continued this pattern of running and walking into the following year. By February 2011, she had lost 100 pounds. So what does one do after losing 100 pounds? She decided to try to run outside. After months of running and walking on the treadmill in her home, she discovered it was much harder to run outside because of the effort and the lack of a controlled environment. But she persevered. In May of that same year, she ran her first non-stop mile. It took 16 minutes. "I was on top of the world," she says.

Jen reached a mental block where she couldn't run more than 3 miles without stopping to walk. A runner friend of hers joined her on a run one day and told her that he would get her over the hump by running with her and encouraging her. "We got to 3 1/2 miles and we high-fived each other!"

A few months later, she signed up for her first 5K race, the Run for Recovery in Watertown, New York. "I woke up that morning and wondered what the heck I was thinking," she says. "But when I arrived at the race, I was shocked that there were people of all shapes and sizes there. There were even some chubby people like me!" She ran the whole distance without stopping. It took her just over 35 minutes. "I was incredibly excited!" she says.

Over time, the pounds melted away, and Jen noticed herself getting stronger and faster. "I challenged myself to run more, to increase my distance," she says. By spring 2012, she was under 150 pounds and running several days per week. Running was part of the new Jen. She ditched the sleep machine that she needed to help her breathe at night. And, despite being told that running would destroy her knees, the pain in her knees was a distant memory. She could easily climb several flights of stairs.

In April 2012, she had surgery to remove the excess skin from her body that resulted from all that lost weight. "I couldn't run while recovering and was really worried I would lose my running fitness," she says. "But I ran as soon as I was cleared to and was thrilled that my body remembered what to do."

In late July, she stepped on the scale and burst into tears. "I weighed 119 pounds, which was my weight-loss goal. I had lost 225 pounds." She admits it wasn't an easy process. "Weight loss isn't linear," she says. "I remember a week when I lost 5 1/2 pounds and there were weeks I lost nothing."

In September, she ran Watertown's Run for Recovery again, but this time she chose the 10K. "It was an out-and-back course, and as I got near the 5K turnaround, I didn't see any women heading back toward me. As I crossed the finish line, I realized that I

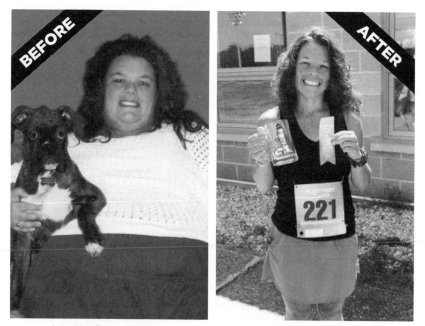

**Jen Hudson Mosher
at 344 pounds.**

**Mosher now,
at 119 pounds.**

had just won a 10K! It was absolutely exhilarating!" Her time was 48:36.

The following May, she ran her first half marathon. And then she ran another. She has run dozens of races, including four half marathons. "When I was 344 pounds, never in a million years would I ever have thought that I could run a 5K, let alone a half marathon," she says. "I sometimes can't even believe that I am the same person."

Despite the enormous weight loss Jen experienced, her journey wasn't without setbacks. In May 2015, she ruptured her Achilles tendon and regained some of the weight during her recovery. And she still is tempted to eat too much. "I believe I have an eating addiction, which I continue to battle," she says. "But I run. It's not as fast or as far as maybe I would like. But running has changed my life. I am a million times happier and healthier than I ever thought possible. I used to be one of those people who said I would never run unless my life depended on it. Now I encourage people who think they can't do it to get out there and start. You don't have to be fast. Anyone can run."

CHAPTER 7

Running and Weight-Loss Myths

"AND THEY WERE SMILING AS THEY FINISHED. THAT WAS ALL IT TOOK."

SHIPPENSBURG UNIVERSITY sits in the rural town of Shippensburg, Pennsylvania, 40 miles southwest of the capital of Harrisburg. If you walk into Shippensburg University's Career and Community Engagement Center, you'll find Assistant Director Sarah McDowell Shupp, a 33-year-old, brown-haired, brown-eyed woman with a big smile who loves Disney and owns a pug named Koda. Overweight for most of her adolescent and adult life, Sarah thought running was something only skinny people did, something one had to be in shape to do. "Any runners I knew were pretty thin and athletic," she says. "I was not."

Growing up, Sarah avoided running or any form of physical activity. The first time she tried to lose weight, she was only 13 years old. She failed. She wasn't any good at team sports or anything athletic and was quickly discouraged from most things she tried. She started to hate all things physical. She was also addicted to food. In high school, she weighed 175 pounds. In college, her weight fluctuated from a high of 202 to a low of 149, but the weight never stayed off. Lack of exercise, poor coping skills, and no boundaries with food led her to a self-imposed 20-year sentence of sitting on the sidelines.

In January 2010, she got involved with a local YMCA's Fitness Challenge, part of which was to run a 5K. She never thought she could run. "The instructor encouraged me to try 2 minutes of running the next time I walked on the treadmill," she says. "So I did. And then I tried 5 minutes. And then 10 minutes. Pretty soon, I was up to 30 minutes of nonstop running on the treadmill."

Then she tried running outside. "It felt terrible and never ending," she remembers. "And God, did I feel slow! I remember running that 5K on a local trail and being so exhausted that I vowed I'd never do it again."

A year later, she met Matthew.

◆ ◆ ◆ ◆ ◆

WHEN I WAS A DOCTORAL STUDENT, my academic advisor would ask me, "Jason, how do you know what you know?" He challenged me to question what I knew and look beyond current dogma to find answers to questions. Like Cicero coining the phrase *"Ipse dixit"* ("He, himself, said it") in reference to the mathematician Pythagoras, we tend to appeal to the pronouncements of the master (in our society, celebrities and the media) rather than to reason or evidence. After all, if Jillian Michaels from TV's *The Biggest Loser* or any other celebrity trainer says it's so, it must be so, right? This has led to the proliferation of many myths in the weight-loss and fitness industry. Why do we think or claim we know things that we actually do not know? There are so many passionate people in the weight-loss and fitness industry, which is great, but oftentimes that passion gets in the way of science. And that can be dangerous. Do you know your running and weight-loss facts from fiction?

MYTH: Running is bad for your knees.

Perhaps the biggest myth about running is that it somehow messes up your knees for life. If I had a nickel for every person who's ever asked me about my knees and commented on running being bad for them, I'd have enough nickels to pay the Kenyans' expensive race appearance fees. Why would an activity humans evolved to do be bad for our bodies? If the activity were harmful to your knees, evolution would have eliminated the ability to run a long time ago because only traits that confer an advantage survive.

People assume that pounding the ground with your legs with so much force must be jarring to your joints. But, if you run correctly, you shouldn't be pounding the ground. You should be rolling through each step, skimming the ground like a pebble on the water, with your body in perfect alignment and your feet landing underneath your hips. Running shouldn't be a jarring activity. When done right, it's smooth and fluid.

> **" PEOPLE WHO RUN HAVE NO GREATER INCIDENCE OF JOINT PROBLEMS OR OSTEOARTHRITIS THAN PEOPLE WHO DON'T RUN."**

Also, the research simply doesn't support that running is bad for your knees. People who run have no greater incidence of joint problems or osteoarthritis than people who don't run. If you have a family history of joint degeneration—if both your parents have had knee replacements or if you already have knee problems when you move a certain way or do certain activities—running can bring that genetic predisposition or those latent issues to the forefront. But running *per se* isn't the underlying cause of your joint problems. As long as you have healthy knees, running isn't bad for them.

MYTH: Your lungs limit your ability to run.

Many new runners complain that they can't breathe as soon as they start running around the block. Indeed, getting enough air is foremost on their minds. It's a marvel of physiology that enough air gets into your body, with your nostrils being no larger than the size of a pea. Even if you run with your mouth half-open, the space is small considering the physiological demand for oxygen at high intensities. A large man who breathes about 0.5 liter of air per breath at rest and about 6 liters of air per minute breathes nearly 200 liters per minute while running hard. That's 53 gallons of air entering the lungs each minute! Try filling a hose with 53 gallons of water in 1 minute. Gives you a lot more respect for the lungs and the effectiveness of diffusion.

At first glance, running seems to have everything to do with big, strong lungs. If the size of your lungs mattered, you'd expect the best runners to have large lungs that hold a lot of air and oxygen. However, the best runners in the world are small compared to the rest of the population, and so they have smaller lungs.

Total lung capacity, which is the maximal amount of air your lungs can hold, is primarily influenced by body size; bigger people have larger lung capacities. I have measured lung capacity in the lab hundreds of times and have found that smaller people have smaller lung capacities, even if they are faster runners.

Despite what you may think or feel when you run, your lungs don't limit your ability, especially if you're not an elite runner. Breathing more deeply to try to get more oxygen in your lungs doesn't make running easier, because oxygen input from the environment doesn't limit your ability to run except when you're running at high altitude. That limitation rests on the shoulders of your cardiovascular and metabolic systems, with blood flow to and oxygen use by your muscles the major culprits. If you're running next to a friend whose breathing is calm and you're huffing and puffing like you're going to blow your house down, that difference is not because your friend has better, bigger lungs. It's because he or she has better (or more trained) cardiovascular and metabolic systems. There's no relationship between your lung capacity and how easy running feels or how fast you run a 10K.

Unlike your cardiovascular and muscular systems, your lungs don't adapt to training. Your lungs do not become "stronger" nor do they become better at sending oxygen to your muscles. The lungs may limit performance only in elite runners who have developed the more trainable characteristics—stroke volume, cardiac output, hemoglobin concentration, and mitochondrial and muscle capillary volumes—to capacities that approach the genetic potential of the lungs to provide for adequate diffusion of oxygen into the blood. In other words, the lungs only become a limiting issue once every other characteristic has been trained to the maximum genetic potential. And this rarely occurs in most runners. Certainly not in beginner runners. The only other instance in which the lungs may limit running is in the case of some kind of diffusion limitation (perhaps because of disease or infection) between the alveoli in the lungs and the pulmonary capillaries, which would hinder the diffusion of oxygen from the lungs into the bloodstream and thus decrease the amount of oxygen transported to your muscles.

When you run at sea level, the main stimulus to breathe is an increase in your blood's carbon dioxide content, not a need for more oxygen. The reason you breathe more when you run faster (or even when you run slow and you're first starting to run) is because carbon dioxide is produced in your muscles from metabolism and needs to be expelled through your lungs. Oxygen is all around you and has no problem diffusing from the air into your lungs. Once inside the lungs, oxygen diffuses into your blood. This elegant process is more than adequate—at sea level, your blood is nearly 100 percent saturated with oxygen, both at rest and even when running as fast as you can. If you run at a high altitude, however, you do breathe more to get more oxygen into your lungs to compensate for your blood being less saturated with oxygen.

Running, which trains your cardiovascular and metabolic characteristics, improves your ability to transport and use oxygen, making you feel less out of breath. So next time you're running up a hill or finishing a hard run and you're thinking, "I can't catch my breath," don't blame your lungs.

MYTH: I'll become scrawny if I run.

Because running is a lower-body exercise, many people think that they'll get scrawny arms by running. Although it's true that running is a much better stimulus for the legs than it is for the arms, your arms are still very active when you run because your upper body must counterbalance the movements of your lower body. Runners typically have defined shoulders because of the repetitive movement of the shoulder to control the arm swing.

Runners come in all shapes and sizes. Not every runner looks like a scrawny Kenyan or Ethiopian. In fact, the only runners who look like the Kenyans and Ethiopians are the Kenyans and Ethiopians. You are not going to become scrawny because you run a few miles every day. Even if you run 50 or more miles per week, you're not going to look scrawny. If you're concerned about getting puny arms, include resistance training a couple of times each week for your upper body.

MYTH: Women shouldn't run while pregnant.

Pregnancy results in profound anatomical and physiological changes that provide nutritional support to the developing fetus and prepare a woman's body for delivery. Although some of these changes can affect a pregnant woman's ability to run, running is actually very good for pregnant women. Almost all women can run up until the third trimester, and many can run through their third trimester. In the absence of either medical or obstetrical complications, pregnant women should do 30 minutes or more of moderate-intensity exercise on most, if not all, days of the week. Aerobic activities like running encourage the flow of blood, oxygen, and nutrients to the developing fetus and can help ease delivery. The frequent complaints of pregnancy, including nausea, heartburn, insomnia, varicose veins, and leg cramps are reduced in women who remain active during their pregnancy. Exercise during pregnancy is also associated with a reduced risk of developing obstetrical complications, including preeclampsia, pregnancy-induced hypertension, and gestational diabetes.

Although running is great for most pregnant women, there are some medical conditions, either pre-existing or that develop during pregnancy, that would prohibit you from running while pregnant. Some of these conditions include heart and lung disease, persistent bleeding in the second and third trimesters, and ruptured membranes. Several other conditions require a careful evaluation of the risks and benefits before continuing with your running program. The most common of these include severe anemia, being extremely underweight, thyroid disease, and inadequate fetal size and development. While these conditions won't necessarily prohibit you from running during your pregnancy, you'll need close monitoring by your doctor.

If you run while pregnant, don't try to set any speed records. Don't increase your mileage or intensity while pregnant, as your body is already under a good deal of stress. Don't try to lose weight (so save this book for after you give birth!). And always discuss your running plans with your doctor.

MYTH: More expensive running shoes are better.

Never be influenced by a shoe's price tag. More expensive doesn't necessarily mean better. There are plenty of great running shoes for less than $100, especially if you buy them at a general sporting goods store instead of a specialty running store. A higher price can mean that the shoe has more technology, or it can simply mean that it's a flashy new model with a high markup price. Most runners don't require all the bells and whistles found in fancy shoe styles. The best shoe for you comes down to what you need for your foot type and running mechanics. Look for a shoe that matches your level of pronation (how much your foot rolls inward when it lands) and feels comfortable right out of the box.

MYTH: Don't run if you have a cold.

Exercise and your immune system have an interesting relationship. Moderate amounts of exercise on a regular basis strengthen your immune system and give you resistance against colds and other upper respiratory tract infections. However, more exercise is not better. Long and intense running can actually weaken your immune system because of the stress it puts on your body. Catching a cold or getting the flu when you run a lot or train for an event like a marathon is very common because your immune system becomes compromised. To help defend against colds and flu, consume both simple and complex carbohydrates (fruits, bread, potatoes, and pasta) as part of your normal diet. Carbohydrate provides energy and also strengthens your immune system by limiting the rise in stress hormones following your workouts.

If you do get sick, here's the golden rule: If the symptoms are above your neck, like a stuffed or runny nose, it's okay to run—just don't try to do a difficult workout or a long run. If the symptoms are below your neck, like a sore throat, coughing, wheezing, or a fever, you shouldn't run. Whether your symptoms are above or below your neck, do what your mother told you—pop some vitamin C, have some chicken soup, drink lots of water, and get plenty of sleep. And stay away from people with colds. If you can't avoid other people, wash your hands throughout the day, especially after shaking someone's hand.

MYTH: Stretching prevents running injuries, reduces soreness, and improves running performance.

Most runners are told that they need to stretch, primarily because running makes your muscles tight and inflexible, and stretching can combat or prevent the inflexibility caused by running. People view inflexibility as a bad thing. But why would running cause an adaptation that is bad for running? All of the other adaptations that running causes are good for running. So why would tight, inflexible muscles be the only adaptation that running causes that is bad for running? That doesn't make sense.

Have you ever run with a dog or watched a horse race? If you have, you probably noticed something interesting—those animals don't stretch before or after they run. When a lion in the wild sees its food running by, it doesn't pause to stretch for a few minutes before chasing after its food. The lion can get up from its lazy, midday nap and immediately chase after a gazelle, and it never gets Achilles tendonitis or iliotibial band syndrome.

Among human animals, stretching attracts a lot of controversy. Although most people have been stretching since their middle school gym class days to prevent injuries, reduce muscle soreness, and improve their ability to run and jump, the research on stretching tells a different story. Despite what your high school gym teacher may have told you, you won't run faster or longer or prevent a running injury just because you bend down to touch your toes before you run.

The research on stretching and injuries is a bit confusing, since there's a lot of conflicting findings. When determining whether stretching reduces injuries, you need to consider the type of activity and type of injury. If the activity includes explosive or bouncing movements, such as volleyball, basketball, and plyometric exercises (exercises that include a lot of jumping and bounding), stretching can reduce injuries by increasing the compliance of your tendons and improve their ability to absorb energy. However, for low-intensity activities that don't include bouncing movements, like running, cycling, and swimming, stretching doesn't prevent injuries because you don't need very compliant tendons for those activities.

In regard to the type of injury, stretching can prevent muscle injuries, such as sprains and strains, but not bone or joint injuries. Bone and joint injuries, which are common among runners, are caused by increasing running mileage or intensity too quickly for your body to adapt.

Stretching before or after you run also has a minimal effect on how sore you feel after your workout. When you exercise harder or longer than you're used to, microscopic damage occurs to your muscle fibers, which is a normal part of exercise. In response to the muscle fiber damage, you get inflammation as more blood travels to the site, bringing with it white blood cells to start the healing process. You feel sore a day or two after a hard workout because of the damage-induced inflammation, which is called *delayed-onset muscle soreness* (DOMS). Stretching doesn't make your muscle fibers heal more quickly, so stretching won't make you feel less sore. Only time and good nutrition, including lots of healthy protein and carbohydrate, reduce soreness as your muscle fibers heal.

Although stretching doesn't reduce the risk of many running-related injuries, reduce muscle soreness in the days after a workout, or improve your running performance, I'm not saying you should never stretch. But there's a time and a place. Stretching can be used to increase mobility and flexibility—a joint's range of motion—thereby priming your muscles to move dynamically through their full ranges of motion, which is important as you age, even if it doesn't directly improve your running or prevent injuries. Flexibility is one of the components of physical fitness. When stretching to increase flexibility, doing it after or apart from your run makes it even more effective.

MYTH: You have to run in your fat-burning zone to burn fat and lose weight.

People often assume that low-intensity exercise is best for burning fat. Cardio equipment manufacturers contribute to this assumption by posting a "fat-burning" workout option on their front panels, which influences people to choose that option because, after all, people want to burn fat. During exercise at a very low intensity, such as walking, fat does account for most of the energy you use. At a moderate intensity, such as running at 80 percent of your maximum heart rate, fat accounts for only about half of the energy you use. While you use both fat and carbohydrate for energy during exercise, these two fuels provide that energy on a sliding scale—as you increase your intensity, the contribution from fat decreases while the contribution from carbohydrate increases. While you use only a minimal amount of fat at faster paces, the number of calories you use per minute and the total number of calories you expend are much greater than when you run at a slower pace, so the amount of fat you use is also greater. Research has shown that the highest rate of fat use occurs when you run at a hard aerobic pace, like the tempo runs described in

Chapters 3 and 4. What matters is the *rate* of energy expenditure rather than simply the percentage of energy expenditure derived from fat. Since you use only carbohydrate when you run at a high intensity, does that mean that if you run fast, you won't get rid of that flabby belly? Of course not.

Despite what most people think, you don't have to use fat when you run to lose fat from your waistline. The little amount of fat that you use in combination with carbohydrate during moderate-intensity exercise is in the form of intramuscular triglycerides—tiny droplets of fat within your muscles. Adipose fat (the fat on your waistline and thighs) is burned during the hours before and after your workouts while you're sitting at your desk. For fat and weight loss, what matters most is the difference between the number of calories you expend and the number of calories you consume. So don't worry about running in your fat-burning zone, because there's no such thing.

MYTH: Running first thing in the morning on an empty stomach burns more fat.

The problem with this myth is that it's true, at least technically. Muscles will indeed use more fat if you run when your blood glucose is low, as it can be first thing in the morning after an overnight fast. But burning more fat during your runs doesn't necessarily mean that you will lose more weight. Running when fasted before breakfast may help you reduce the total number of calories you consume throughout the day, but it doesn't allow you to cheat the laws of caloric balance; at the end of the day, you still have to have a caloric deficit to lose fat.

When you run first thing in the morning before breakfast, your muscles don't just rely on fat immediately. When running at a slow or moderate pace, they'll use some fat, just like they would when you run at any other time of the day. But they'll also use whatever carbohydrate is available from blood glucose and stored glycogen because carbohydrate is the muscles' preferred fuel. When you run out of glucose, your muscles will then start to rely more heavily on fat. But running on an empty stomach with low blood glucose decreases the intensity at which you can run, which results in a lower-quality workout and less total calories burned. For weight loss, it really doesn't matter if the calories you burn when you run come from fat or carbohydrate; how many *total calories* you burn when you run is what matters.

If you have a light breakfast containing carbohydrate of about 200 to 300 calories about 30 to 60 minutes before you run, you'll feel better and have a higher-quality workout, which will ultimately help you burn more calories. If you can't wait that long, consume something easily digestible, like a banana or a slice of toast with peanut butter.

MYTH: Muscle weighs more than fat.

Like the riddle many of us have been asked—Which weighs more: a pound of feathers or a pound of gold?—muscle and fat weigh exactly the same. A pound of muscle is equal to a pound of fat. The difference between muscle and fat is the same difference as between feathers and gold—their densities. Muscle is denser than fat because it has less volume for its mass (density = mass ÷ volume). That means that 5 pounds of muscle take up less room on your body (and look better) than do 5 pounds of fat. Unfortunately, it's much easier to put on 5 pounds of fat than it is to put on 5 pounds of muscle.

MYTH: Doing sit-ups and crunches will shrink your waistline.

If you stay up until one or two in the morning and flip through the channels on your television, you'll likely come across an infomercial touting the newest way to get a flat stomach and six-pack abs. Unfortunately, sit-ups and crunches, regardless of how and on what fancy equipment they are done, will not shrink your waistline. Since you have to expend about 3,500 calories more than you consume to lose 1 pound, it would take probably a million crunches to add up to enough calories to make a difference in the size of your waistline. Crunches and other core exercises can strengthen your abdominal muscles, but they won't make you lose the fat covering them. The flat stomachs and six-pack abs on the models in those infomercials or in print ads in magazines didn't get that way from whatever abdominal exercise gadget the infomercial or advertisement is selling. They got that way from having great genes and from doing other types of exercise that burn many calories (and from airbrushing print images). Those "visual testimonials" are just clever marketing.

MYTH: Each pound of muscle burns 50 calories per day.

Unfortunately, muscle doesn't burn nearly as many calories per day as most people think. Research using body imaging techniques such as MRI and PET scans to calculate organ surface area and energy cost has shown that each pound of muscle burns about 6 to 7 calories per day. Even as far back as 1971, scientists calculated that resting metabolic rate in children and adolescents was equal to 8 calories per pound of muscle per day. By contrast, each pound of fat burns 2 to 3 calories per day, so while muscle does burn more calories than fat, the difference is very small. If you were to add 5 pounds of muscle to your body (which would take months of specific resistance training), you'll burn only about 30 to 35 more calories per day at rest. That's about as many calories as one-third of a glass of milk. The extra muscle can become valuable when you run, because you'll have more muscle engaged in—and therefore more calories burned during—the activity.

MYTH: Resistance training increases resting metabolic rate.

I often hear personal trainers tell their weight-loss clients that they have to do resistance training to increase muscle mass because muscles are "fat-burning machines." If you want to lose weight, they say, the increase in resting metabolic rate will help you burn more calories all day. Perhaps the biggest myth in the fitness industry is the issue of resistance training increasing resting metabolic rate by increasing muscle mass, which leads to greater weight loss. Although it is true that resting metabolic rate is influenced by the amount of muscle you have, you would have to add a lot of muscle to significantly impact your resting metabolic rate. It's not like you can add 10 pounds of muscle (which is very difficult to do unless you train like a bodybuilder for many months) and all of a sudden your resting metabolic rate is double what it was before. Most research shows about a 10-calorie increase in metabolic rate for every pound of muscle. So, if your resting metabolic rate is 1,500 calories per day, you would need to add 15 pounds of muscle mass to increase it by 10 percent. Resistance training can make you look better because of the effect it has on your muscles, but it won't really impact your resting metabolic rate much. As you lose weight, your resting metabolic rate actually decreases, even when you maintain muscle mass by resistance training. Some research has shown that exercise can prevent the decline in resting metabolic rate as you lose weight, but no research shows that resting metabolic rate *increases* as you lose weight.

As mentioned in Chapter 2, humans' resting metabolic rate—the amount of energy you need to stay alive—is pretty stable, having been set by millions of years of evolution. Lifting dumb-bells in a gym or doing burpees in the park is not going to change that. Research *has* shown that metabolic rate can be acutely raised in the hours after a workout while you recover, especially if the workout is long and/or hard. However, an increased resting metabolic rate is not a chronic adaptation to exercise training. Some studies have shown an increase in resting metabolic rate following many weeks or months of exercise, but the magnitude of change is relatively small (about 30 to 142 calories per day) compared to what is needed for weight loss. And some of these studies have been done on seniors, who are more likely to show increases in resting metabolic rate due to the attenuating effect of exercise on age-associated losses in muscle mass. It's much easier to impact muscle mass and thus resting metabolic rate in an older person than in a younger person.

MYTH: Intense workouts contribute to weight loss by burning more calories after the workout is over.

Ever since the fitness industry found research showing that people burn calories after they work out while they recover from their workout, a whole new argument was born. Exercise stopped being about the exercise and became about what came after. "Do this workout," trainers and gurus would say, "because you'll burn four times as many calories for up to 48 hours afterward."

Oh, if burning calories and losing weight were only that easy. After some workouts, specifically those that are intense or long, you continue to use oxygen and burn calories because you must recover from the workout, and recovery is an aerobic, oxygen-using process. This increased oxygen consumption following the workout is called the *excess postexercise oxygen consumption* (EPOC).

Many studies have documented the EPOC and compared it and its associated postworkout calorie burn between exercise of different intensities and durations. However, the postworkout calorie burn caused by the EPOC is a highly overexaggerated issue among fitness trainers. The increase in metabolism is transient, perhaps lasting a few hours, depending on how intense the workout was. The unbridled optimism regarding the EPOC in weight loss is generally unfounded. Studies have shown that the EPOC comprises only 6 to 15 percent of the net total oxygen cost of the exercise, and only when the exercise is very intense. Since unfit individuals recover more slowly than fit individuals, the EPOC will be higher in unfit individuals. However, most unfit individuals simply can't handle the intensity of exercise that is required to induce a high or prolonged EPOC.

> **"THE CALORIES YOU BURN WHEN YOU RUN HAVE A GREATER EFFECT ON YOUR BODY WEIGHT THAN THE CALORIES YOU BURN AFTERWARD. IT IS THE RUN ITSELF THAT CREATES THE DEMAND FOR CHANGE."**

The calories you burn when you run have a greater effect on your body weight than the calories you burn afterward. It is the run itself that creates the demand for change.

MYTH: Thin people have a faster metabolism.

Try this experiment: Hold five copies of this book in one hand and one copy in the other. Which arm is doing more work to hold the books? In which arm is metabolic rate faster?

Did you answer correctly? Just because I'm thin doesn't mean I have a fast metabolism. Heavier people actually have a faster metabolism because it takes more energy to support a heavier weight than it does to support a lighter weight, just like holding five copies of this book in your hand takes more energy than holding one copy.

When it comes to expending energy, body weight matters. As Isaac Newton's second law of motion (the Law of Acceleration) tells us, an acceleration is produced when a force acts on an object and is equal to that force divided by the object's mass ($a = F \div m$, or its more recognized form, $F = m \times a$). The greater the object's mass, the more force is required to get it moving. This is why a heavy person uses more calories doing the same exercise at the same intensity than does a light person.

MYTH: Eating multiple small meals throughout the day rather than three large meals is better for weight loss.

Many weight-loss proponents suggest that eating multiple small meals throughout the day is better than eating only breakfast, lunch, and dinner. Practically speaking, it may be a good idea to eat more often throughout the day to prevent an empty stomach. However, research hasn't shown that eating more often decreases appetite. The handful of research studies on meal frequency does not support that it enhances diet-induced thermogenesis (the caloric cost of digestion), total energy expenditure, or resting metabolic rate, or that it plays a significant role in decreasing body weight or body composition. For weight loss, it seems that eating a specific number of calories in three meals or in six meals doesn't matter. So feel free to eat multiple smaller meals each day if that's what's convenient, as long as your total calories for the day stay in check.

MYTH: Eating right before going to bed will make you fat.

Most nights, a few hours after dinner, I eat a bowl of cereal. If I eat the cereal at 7:59 p.m., I never gain weight. But if I eat the cereal at 8:01 p.m., it goes right to my hips and thighs. See how silly that sounds? The enzymes that break down food and are responsible for storing fat don't wear watches. The only reason why eating before going to bed may increase your chance of gaining weight is because of the greater number of daily calories that results from eating at night, not the actual time on the clock. People tend to snack at night while watching television with their families, which means eating more calories. If you create a metabolic demand throughout the day by running a lot and doing other forms of exercise, the calories you consume, regardless of whether you consume them 1 hour before going to bed or 3 hours before going to bed, will be used to meet the metabolic demand and not get stored as fat.

MYTH: Low-carb diets help you lose weight.

There actually is some truth to this myth. Research shows that low-carb diets can and do result in rapid weight loss. So if your goal is to lose weight in the next few weeks because you have an event to go to and want to look good, then cutting out most (but not all) of the carbs from your diet will help you lose weight fast. However, not all studies have found that low-carb diets are more effective for weight loss than moderate- or high-carb diets. And low-carb diets, while popular, are probably not good for the long term because they are not a sustainable strategy. Can you go the rest of your life on a low-carb diet? Probably not, especially if you run a lot. Personally, I have never met a runner on a low-carb diet for more than a short term. Most weight-loss studies are of short duration, leaving little research on the long-term effects of a low-carb diet on exercise and weight loss. You need to exercise to keep the weight off, and carbohydrate is the muscles' preferred fuel during exercise. Without adequate carbohydrate in your muscles and blood, your workouts will likely suffer and you probably won't feel good during them. Carbs are also important to keep your immune system strong so you don't get sick; and, from a biochemical standpoint, you need an adequate supply of carbs for fat to be burned effectively because fat burns in the flame of carbohydrate. If you consume a low-carb diet, there's not much carbohydrate available in your muscles, so your body makes metabolic adaptations to shift metabolism toward a greater reliance on fat during low-intensity exercise. This may be a good thing for low-intensity exercise, but high-intensity workouts require carbohydrate for energy.

MYTH: Nutrition (diet) is more important than exercise for losing weight and looking good.

I hear a lot in the fitness industry about the importance of clean eating. Indeed, most fitness professionals quote that physical appearance is 80 percent due to nutrition and 20 percent due to your workouts. I don't know where those numbers come from, but those percentages are unknowable.

If we are to assign a relative importance to each, it's presumptuous to think that the specific foods we eat are more important to our health, fitness, and cosmetics than are genetics and training. People like to claim that abs are made in the kitchen, but the truth is that muscles—at least those of your lower body—are made by running and other types of exercise. I'm pretty sure I didn't get my sculpted legs and ass from eating kale salads; I got them from running 6 days per week for 33 years. And so it is for other runners as well.

This is not to say that a person's diet doesn't matter. Of course it does. But to place such a large emphasis on diet over exercise misses an important point—cutting calories and eating a more nutritious diet does not make you fitter. Although your nutrition is undoubtedly important, it doesn't give your muscles a stimulus to adapt. Only exercise can do that and thus give you all of the fitness and health benefits. The sculpted legs of runners and upper bodies of fitness magazine models didn't get that way just by eating fruits and vegetables.

Research shows that you need both diet *and* exercise. Diet gets your weight off, especially initially, and exercise keeps it off. To lose weight, you must consume fewer calories each day. To maintain weight, you must exercise on most, if not all, days of the week. There is a ton of research to show that body weight and body mass index are directly proportional to the amount of exercise people do.

If we take two people, and one eats perfectly clean with a nutrient-dense diet and no processed foods but doesn't exercise much, and the other runs a lot and does resistance training but has a mediocre diet with the occasional Twinkie or chocolate chip cookie, who is going to look better and be fitter? I hope you said the latter. Truth is, exercise and genetics exert a greater influence on how you look (and on your physical performance) than your diet does.

MYTH: Small, sustained changes in energy intake or expenditure will produce large, long-term weight changes.

People are often told to park at the far end of the parking lot and take the stairs instead of the elevator. Ever wonder if these strategies really work? Although every calorie matters when you're trying to lose weight, unfortunately, parking your car farther away from the entrance of the store and taking the stairs instead of the elevator are not going to have as large of an impact as you want. The extra calories you'll burn by parking 1,000 feet from the store instead of 200 feet are negligible. For most people, these small lifestyle changes are easily compensated for by their diet. However, these lifestyle behaviors get you in the habit of being more active throughout the day. And that's a good thing.

MYTH: There's a magical combination of foods or a specific diet that is most effective for weight loss.

Although every weight-loss book author likes to believe that his or her diet is better than every other diet on the market, there isn't any scientific evidence that one particular diet will work better with an individual's specific metabolism. Your metabolism isn't even all that unique. Biologically, humans are much more alike than they are different. The reason the best diet myth sticks around is almost certainly because of how much money there is to be made off of it. The weight-loss industry is a multibillion dollar industry. Any diet will help you lose weight if you follow it and stick to it. There's no magic diet. The truth is that all diets, if they limit calories and are combined with exercise, work if you follow and stick with them.

" THE TRUTH IS THAT ALL DIETS, IF THEY LIMIT CALORIES AND ARE COMBINED WITH EXERCISE, WORK IF YOU FOLLOW AND STICK WITH THEM."

♦ ♦ ♦ ♦ ♦

IN MAY 2011, Sarah McDowell Shupp started dating Matthew, now her husband, who asked her to accompany him to a half marathon he was running in Philadelphia. At that time, she had been running for a year and a half, mainly to try to lose weight, with little success. "It wasn't something I really enjoyed," she says. "It was more of a means to an end rather than a lifestyle change."

But something changed for her while watching the half marathon.

"As I stood at the finish line and watched people finish the race, I was shocked to see people who looked overweight and not athletic like me," she says. "And they were smiling as they finished. That was all it took. I was so completely inspired that I signed up for a 5K in my hometown right from my cell phone while I was watching the finishers from that half marathon. I ran my first 5K the next month and was hooked on the energy of organized races. Since then, I've run countless 5Ks and 10Ks, 17 half marathons, and 2 marathons.

Since she made the commitment to lose weight, Sarah lost 50 pounds in 26 months. She blogs about her running and weight loss at sparklyrunner.com. She now maintains her weight between 140 and 146 pounds. "Losing weight was incredibly difficult," she says. "I spent 30 years creating horrible eating habits for myself and it was hard to change those habits." She pauses. "It's still difficult. It's probably harder to maintain a healthy weight than it is to lose weight.

"I've learned that staying active—especially running—is key to keeping the weight off," Sarah says. "But I've also learned that just because I run doesn't mean I can eat whatever I want. In fact, it's the opposite. I was running 40 miles per week and was still about 30 pounds overweight because I wasn't paying attention to what I was eating. In my experience, runners often overestimate how many calories they've burned during a run and they tend to overcompensate and eat more than they would had they not run. When I'm in the midst of training, I need to eat lean and clean: lots of unprocessed, natural food—mostly lean proteins, fruits, and vegetables. Eating crap makes my running crap." To support her weight-loss goals, Sarah joined the Weight Watchers program.

"Living healthy has become my new normal," Sarah says, "but old habits are hard to break. I still reach for comfort food and still make unhealthy decisions when I'm tired or frustrated." But the majority of the time, Sarah has learned to make other choices. "I've learned to focus on the benefits of healthy choices, not on the sacrifice of giving up the comforting but unhealthy foods."

In addition to her job in the career center at Shippensburg University, Sarah now works part-time for the company that helped her lose weight. She facilitates the Weight Watchers' members' weigh-ins, processes payments for product purchases, and carries out other administrative duties. She is currently in training

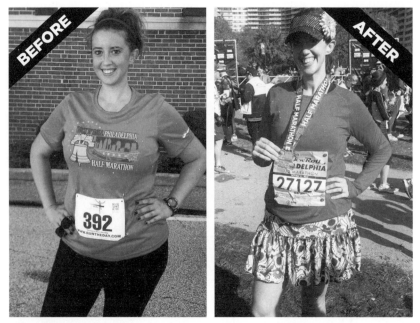

Sarah McDowell Shupp, whose heaviest weight was 202 pounds.

Shupp now, at 140 pounds.

to become a Weight Watchers leader so she can have an even greater impact by leading the members' weekly meetings.

When I asked Sarah what advice she has for others who are trying to lose weight, she says, "Make small changes slowly. It's unrealistic to radically change your diet overnight and expect that to be a lasting change. You have to view losing weight and getting healthy as a true change in your lifestyle. Don't make any changes that you can't live with forever. If you view losing weight as only having to do it for a certain amount of time, your results will be temporary."

Sarah races nearly every weekend, often in sparkly outfits. "Running has truly changed my life in the most astounding ways," she says. "I've learned that I am worth taking care of and the best way to do that is to eat healthy foods and move as much as possible. The positive energy, constant encouragement, and unwavering support shown by the running community has kept me running for the last 3 years and helped me complete over 90 races. It is my sincere hope that I can inspire others to do something amazing and impossible."

CHAPTER 8

Preventing Running Injuries

**"I BROKE MY FOOT WHILE TRAINING
FOR MY FIRST MARATHON BY STEPPING ON A WALNUT."**

THE 2016 BOSTON MARATHON was only 6 weeks after Mark Falkingham's 3-year anniversary. Standing on the start line at 5-foot-6 and 156 pounds with muscular calves, Mark looks like a runner. He sounds like one, too—his Facebook page is filled with daily posts about running, and most of his Facebook friends are runners talking up their runs. But Mark didn't always look or sound this way.

On March 1, 2013, Mark's health was a mess. He weighed 269 pounds and had type 2 diabetes, sleep apnea, high blood pressure, and high cholesterol. He wasn't running a step. He grew up in Canada, drinking beer and playing hockey like most good Canadian boys. As he entered his late teens, the hockey stopped, but the beer continued into his 20s, when he discovered his love for food, especially fatty and fried food. "You know, the really tasty kind," the self-proclaimed food addict says. His running partner tells him that she loves to watch him eat because it's like he's making love to the food.

After moving to Aurora, Illinois, Mark continued his love affair with food and was sedentary into his late 30s. "The next thing I knew, I was over 200 pounds," he says. At age 38, he began an online gaming obsession. He spent nearly 11 years sitting on his butt, playing Everquest; eating chips, cheeseburgers, and fries; drinking beer and soda; and smoking two packs of cigarettes per day. His average lunch was two double-quarter-pound cheeseburgers, large fries, 10 chicken nuggets, and a large chocolate milkshake.

"I was lazy and didn't care about my appearance or my health," he says. "I didn't think I was going to get sick from this. I was just doing what most other people do, so how could this be bad? I was not educated about obesity, eating, smoking, and drinking. I just thought it was normal."

But with all of his health issues, Mark knew he had to make a change. "With my wife's help, all of the food in the house was loaded into two giant trash bags and tossed out," he says. He started working out at a gym the next day, doing mostly cardio exercises mixed with weight machines.

After 3 months, his weight down 54 pounds, he hit a plateau. "I got on the treadmill and couldn't run 3 minutes," he says, "which made me want to figure out how to do more." He worked his way up to 5 minutes, then 7, then 10, 15, and 30 minutes. After 6 months, he had lost 100 pounds and his doctor declared him free of diabetes and sleep apnea. His blood pressure and cholesterol were perfect, and he was running nonstop for 1 hour on the treadmill.

One day, someone at the gym mentioned to him that he had the wrong shoes for running and that he should have his gait analyzed, so he visited a local running specialty store to have his gait checked and to buy real running shoes. While in the store, Mark saw a brochure for a Walk 2 Run program—10 weeks from walking to running a 5K. He signed up for it.

◆ ◆ ◆ ◆ ◆

WHEN I WAS IN HIGH SCHOOL, my electronics teacher had a silly saying to remind his students of how to handle electrical wires: "One hand in pockey, no get shockey." Like touching wires with both hands, there's a wrong way to do almost everything. For example, throwing a paper airplane at your high school teacher, wearing leg warmers on the treadmill, and not buying your twin brother a birthday present—claiming you forgot his birthday—would all be considered by most as errors in judgment. (Okay, so I don't always make the best decisions.) Although starting and continuing a running program the wrong way may not have as severe a consequence as electrocuting yourself, it can cause you to injure yourself. Since you can't run to burn calories when you're injured, that's a severe enough consequence if you're trying to lose weight.

I'm proud to say that in all my years of running, I've never had a running-related injury. However, for the majority of runners, it's a different story. Beginning runners often get injured because they haven't yet run enough to strengthen their anatomy to withstand the stress of running. And the longer you're a runner, the more likely you are to get injured because the more years you subject your body to the stress of the activity.

At least half of all runners deal with at least one injury per year, and 25 percent of runners are injured at any given time. But injuries don't have to be an inevitable part of running. Sometimes you can get injured no matter how careful you are, but the secrets in this chapter will get you darn close to preventing any running injuries.

Most injuries happen because the physical stress from running is too much for your body to handle at that time. The human body is great at adapting to stress, but only when you apply it in small doses. When you apply the stress too quickly for your body to adapt, something breaks down. This is especially true with running, because running imposes a force of two to three times your body weight on each leg with each step.

The causes of running injuries can be divided into intrinsic factors (which are specific to you) and extrinsic factors (which are related to your training and environment).

Intrinsic factors include:

◆ **Previous injury:** The single biggest intrinsic predictor of injury is previous injury. Already having an injury shows that that body part is vulnerable.

◆ **Age:** Older runners are more susceptible to injuries because they take longer to recover from workouts and adapt to the training.

◆ **Sex:** Female runners often have a greater risk of injury than do male runners. The wider hips of females cause the femur bone to meet the patella at an angle, which can cause the patella to move laterally within its groove, increasing a woman's chance of knee injury. Also, irregular menstrual cycles and menopause cause a drop in or even an absence of the hormone that protects women's bones—estrogen. Females' bones are less dense than males' bones to begin with, so their bones are more susceptible to injury.

◆ **Bone density:** Low bone density increases the risk of stress fractures.

◆ **Lack of running experience:** If you're a new runner, you have a greater risk of injury because you're not yet used to the stress of running.

◆ **Foot type:** Flat feet that pronate (roll inward) excessively when you run can cause injuries because flat feet are more susceptible to overpronation.

Extrinsic factors include:

◆ **Running volume:** How many miles you run per week is the greatest extrinsic predictor of injury risk. It's hard to say exactly how many miles per week increases the risk of injury, because that's an individual matter. You may be able to handle 40 miles per week, and your running partner may get injured with 20. Some runners (called Olympians) can run more than 100 miles per week and not get injured! On average, the risk of getting injured is two to three times greater when running at least 40 miles per week.

◆ **Intensity:** Running at a faster pace, such as when doing interval workouts, places a greater stress on your legs.

◆ **Shoes:** Running in the wrong shoes can adversely affect lower-extremity alignment, making you more susceptible to injury. For instance, a cushioning shoe isn't a good choice for an overpronator, who needs a shoe that offers more stability. Anytime you get a running-related injury, that's a good sign to change your shoes, usually to a different type.

For all running-related injuries, focus your treatment on the underlying cause rather than on the symptoms. If you focus on the symptoms, you may feel better, but you won't eliminate the reason why the injury happened in the first place.

Injuries don't *have* to be a part of running. They happen because of unintelligent training, by doing too much too soon. Imagine if a bridge were poorly engineered. Wouldn't it be at risk for breaking down? If you train smart by following the secrets in this chapter, I can almost guarantee that you won't get injured, and you'll run healthier and better for it.

SECRET #1: Train intelligently.

The number one reason why runners get injured is because they're not smart about how they train. To train intelligently, optimize your workouts so you run at more effective levels of effort to get the best results. You want to obtain the greatest benefit while incurring the least amount of stress. How do you do that? Run only as fast as you need to in order to obtain the result you desire. The goal of running is not to run as fast or as hard or as long as you can every time you head out the door; that will just exhaust you. Even when you run faster, like during an interval workout, you want to control your pace to get the most out of it. The *Run Your Fat Off* program is designed to help you train intelligently; if you follow it closely, you're not likely to overdo it and get injured.

SECRET #2: Increase your running volume very slowly and spread it out over the whole week.

The slower you increase your weekly volume, the less chance you'll get injured. When you increase the amount of running you do, add only about 0.5 mile to 1 mile (about 5 to 10 minutes) per day of running so that you spread the stress around. For example, if you currently run 10 miles in 3 days per week, run no more than 13 miles next week by adding 1 mile to each of the 3 days. Don't run 13 miles next week by adding all 3 miles to only 1 day of running. Many popular magazines and websites, such as *Runner's World* and *Women's Running*, as well as many runners and coaches, quote a 10 percent rule of increasing mileage, but there's nothing special about 10 percent. You can often increase by more than that if you're smart about how you do it.

> **"RUN ONLY AS FAST AS YOU NEED TO IN ORDER TO OBTAIN THE RESULT YOU DESIRE."**

If you've already been running and are pretty fit, you may be able to get away with adding more miles more quickly, especially if you have experience running more miles. For example, if you've run 40 miles per week in the recent past and now you're training for your fifth half marathon and building your mileage, you don't necessarily have to go from 20 to 25 to 30 to 35 to 40 miles per week over a couple of months. You may be able to make bigger jumps in mileage because your legs already have experience running 40 miles per week. However, if 40 miles per week is brand-new territory for you, then you do need to increase your mileage in smaller increments. Again, if you follow the *Run Your Fat Off* program, you'll see that you are increasing your mileage gradually with each course.

SECRET #3: Don't increase your running volume every week.

If you're a new runner, an older runner, or are prone to injury, run the same mileage for 2 to 4 weeks before increasing it. Give your legs a chance to fully absorb and adapt to the workload before increasing the workload. You want 10 miles per week to be a normal experience for your body before increasing to 15 miles per week. And that takes time. You'll see in the *Run Your Fat Off* menus that the running mileage increases with each course, so spend 2 to 4 weeks in each course before moving on to the next.

SECRET #4: Don't increase the distance of your long run every week.

This is especially important if you're entering uncharted territory with your long runs (i.e., you've never run that distance or for that length of time before). Repeat the same long run for a few weeks before running longer. You want a 6-mile run to become normal before you try to run 7 miles. Ramping up the long run too quickly is a good way for new or recreational runners to get injured, since you would be increasing the stress week after week after week.

SECRET #5: Don't make your long run too long.

Don't make your long run more than about a third of your weekly volume of running. If you are running 21 miles per week, for instance, your long run should be no more than 7 miles. The point is to not accumulate too much stress in one run. Don't misunderstand—the long run should be stressful. After all, you're running for a long time, burning a lot of calories, and trying to make yourself tired so your body adapts. However, it's better to spread the stress around. If you're only able to run a few days per week, though, it may be hard to stick to this rule. If your long run winds up being a lot more than a third of your weekly mileage, do a midweek, medium-long run that's about 65 to 75 percent of the length (or duration) of your long run. This way, your long run isn't so much more stressful than other runs during the week, which reduces the injury risk.

SECRET #6: Take a step back before taking two steps forward.

Every few weeks, decrease your weekly running volume by about a third for 1 recovery week to give your legs a chance to absorb and respond to the training you've done. For example, if you've run 20 miles per week for the last 3 weeks, back off to 13 miles for 1 week before increasing above 20 miles for the next week. You'll notice the difference it makes in how your legs feel, and you'll start the week after the recovery week on fresh legs that are capable of handling more work.

SECRET #7: Don't increase your weekly volume and the intensity of your workouts at the same time.

Your legs can handle only so much stress at once. When you begin to include interval workouts in your running program, don't try to add time to your runs that week. You might even want to run a little bit less in the first week or two. Trying to increase how much you run while also increasing the intensity of your workouts is too much for most people to handle. The *Run Your Fat Off* menus take a methodical approach to increasing volume and intensity, with the weekly volume only increasing a little at a time when the intensity is already increased. This is why it is imperative that you repeat each week of each course multiple times before moving on to the next course.

SECRET #8: Alternate hard days and easy days.

Every day you do a harder workout, whether it be running related or even another form of exercise, follow it with at least 1 day of easy running. Don't run hard more than 2 to 3 days per week.

SECRET #9: Run easy on your easy days.

By running too fast on your easy days, you add unnecessary stress to your legs without any extra benefit. You also won't be able to run more over time, which burns more calories, and you won't be able to handle more intense workouts on other days, which are important to boost fitness and burn even more calories. Easy runs should feel gentle and allow you to hold a conversation, even if that conversation is with yourself (sometimes that's the best conversation to have). Initially, even slow runs are hard if you're overweight and haven't run before. But don't worry; that will change.

SECRET #10: Train appropriately for you.

Running with others can be really motivating and helpful, but unless you are at a similar fitness level and at the same point in your running programs, don't just follow what they do. If your friend Jason is running 5 miles on Saturday but the longest you've run is 2 miles, don't try to run the whole 5 miles with him. It's okay and even beneficial to run with people who are a little bit faster and fitter so they can push you to be better

> **"ALL ADAPTATIONS TO RUNNING OCCUR WHILE YOU'RE RECOVERING FROM YOUR RUNS, NOT WHILE YOU'RE RUNNING."**

yourself. But don't do that too often or you may get run into the ground and get injured.

SECRET #11: Get adequate recovery.

All adaptations to running occur while you're recovering from your runs, not while you're running. If you adequately recover between runs, your muscles, bones, tendons, and ligaments won't break down. The older you are, the more time you need to recover, so give yourself more time between harder days of running and before increasing your weekly running volume and intensity. This means you may need to slightly modify the *Run Your Fat Off* running menus to add more easy days and stick with each course for 3 or 4 or maybe even more weeks before moving on to the next course.

Time is the most influential part of recovery. However, nutrition, hydration, the amount of activity you do the rest of the day, and sleep all affect recovery. So pay attention to all of those things.

SECRET #12: Reduce overpronation.

Because overpronation—when your foot rolls inward too much upon landing on the ground—is a common cause of many running-related injuries, try to reduce any pronation that is more than normal. Wear the correct type of shoes for your feet and running mechanics (e.g., cushioning/neutral, stability, or motion-control shoes); limit running on roads that are cambered (or slanted) near the gutter for rainwater drainage, which increases ankle pronation of the outside foot; and strengthen your calves with resistance exercises to help stabilize your lower leg when it lands on the ground.

SECRET #13: Balance strength imbalances.

When muscles are weak, other muscles and tendons must absorb more of the stress of running. If you're a beginner runner who hasn't exercised much before reading this book, chances are you have some weak areas. Even intermediate or advanced runners can be weak if they've only been training a specific way. Targeted resistance training can help eliminate muscle strength imbalances and thus protect tendons and joints from injury. Eccentric resistance training, during which muscles are forced to lengthen under tension, like when you lower a heavy weight, is very effective for increasing muscle strength. You are only as strong as your weakest link; strengthen your weakest link and you'll run better and healthier!

◆ ◆ ◆ ◆ ◆

AFTER 10 WEEKS, the Walk 2 Run program Mark Falkingham had joined concluded with the Tails 5K9 in De Kalb, Illinois, organized by a local animal shelter. He completed the race without a problem. "I was a little ahead of the curve and very motivated to do more—to run harder and faster and to keep finding my limits."

So Mark set his sights—and his legs—on longer races. During his first year as a runner, he planned to run four half marathons and a full marathon, but a walnut thwarted part of his plan. "I ran three half marathons and broke my foot by stepping on a walnut while training for my first marathon," he says. "I was out 10 weeks, missed my first marathon, and was devastated."

After 10 weeks, Mark's doctor cleared him to run. Six weeks later, Mark ran a half marathon and, a week after that, he ran a 50K (31 miles) because "I needed to run 26.2 miles or more to make up for missing my first full marathon," he says.

When I spoke to Mark, a process and applications engineer, he was getting ready to run another 50K. He had already run nine half marathons, three marathons, qualified for the 2016 Boston Marathon, and ran a 50-mile ultramarathon, in which he won the 50- to 59-year-old age group and placed eighth overall in 7 hours, 57 minutes. "I'm extremely motivated to stay healthy and see what my body is capable of at 51 years of age," he says. "I've learned that I can do anything I set my mind to and that I am stronger than I had given myself credit for."

To date, Mark has lost a total of 113 pounds. "To lose that much weight in 6 months might make it seem easy, but it wasn't," he says. "It was one of the hardest things I have ever done. It took a 150 percent commitment—no cheats, no treats, no slacking off. Nothing but hard work and dedication. You have to want to do it in your head but also in your heart. If you don't want to do this in both places, it is doomed to failure.

"Weight loss is really hard. It requires a significantly strong person, and combining it with an endurance sport such as running means you are working hard, struggling with two things at the same time. Running for me is about pushing myself, pushing envelopes, finding out what I am made of, how far I can go, how long I can go, how fast I can go. I'm having a great time with this."

If only there were more people like Mark Falkingham.

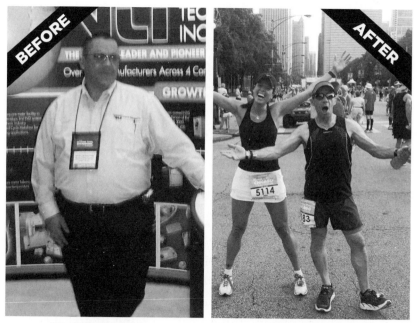

**Mark Falkingham
at 269 pounds.**

**Falkingham now,
at 156 pounds.**

COOL-DOWN

WHEN I SET OUT TO WRITE a weight-loss book, I had no idea where it was going to take me. I wanted to blend the scientific research with the real-life stories of people who have lost weight through running, and do that with enough inspiration to get people off their couches and running. For the most part, I knew what I wanted to say, but I didn't know the impact that writing such a book would have on me. All along I thought I was the one providing the inspiration, but after reading the people's stories woven throughout this book, I realized they are the ones who provide the inspiration. None of these people thought they could be runners when they were fat and out of shape. Certainly none of them thought about running a half marathon or marathon. Had you suggested they could run around the block, they would have laughed at that notion. But they did run. They didn't follow any particular diet, such as Atkins, Paleo, or celebrity-endorsed cleanse. They just ran and consumed fewer calories. And they transformed their lives. They became runners. They became marathoners. They became Ironman triathletes.

That these people began to run races and continued to run races throughout their weight-loss journey reveals the pull that running has. It pulls us in a direction that no other exercise does. And that's why running is the best exercise for weight loss—because running doesn't just change you physically; it changes you psychologically and emotionally. It is for these reasons that you'll keep running—and maintain your weight—for the rest of your life. These people are perfect examples of what you can accomplish when you put your mind to it and imagine a better life for yourself. Even this lifelong runner is inspired by their accomplishments and their ability to change.

You don't have to run marathons or ultramarathons to lose weight. You just need to start running—and keep running. And wherever that running takes you is up to you. When you throw yourself into running to lose weight, clear of the doubts that hold you back, the payoff is extraordinary no matter what the scale in your bathroom reads. But if you stick with running, that scale will read lighter and, perhaps even more important, your life will be changed forever. And that is worth the price of enough pairs of running shoes to last the rest of your slimmer and healthier life.

APPENDIX A: CHOOSING RUNNING SHOES

YOU TAKE APPROXIMATELY **1,000 STEPS** with each foot every mile you run, so you want every one of those steps to be as comfortable as possible. There seems to be a lot of confusion about which shoes runners should wear. From the "minimalist" Vibram Five Finger shoes that have no cushioning at all and mimic running barefoot to the "maximalist" HOKA One One shoes that have lots of cushioning, there is no shortage of running shoes on the market. With all of the different types and all of their bells and whistles, how do you know what you need? The choice depends on what feels comfortable, the amount of cushioning or support you need, how much you run, and how much your foot pronates when it lands on the ground.

When you walk into a running shoe store, the array of shoes can be dizzying. Despite the large selection, there really aren't as many shoes as it seems. Fewer types of shoes exist than do types of toothpaste.

Running shoes have specific combinations of cushioning and support designed for the varying degrees of pronation and comfort among runners. Shoes are divided by the manufacturers into three major categories: cushioning/neutral, stability, and motion control. Other shoes are designed for specific running conditions, such as trail running and racing. The shoes are usually labeled by category in running shoe stores.

Most runners' feet make contact with the ground with the outside part of the heel. The foot then rolls inward (pronates) to absorb shock and optimally distribute the forces of impact. With the whole foot on the ground through the stance phase, the entire ball of the foot is used to push off the ground. How much you pronate largely dictates the choice of running shoes. Most runners pronate just enough for the foot to absorb shock and thus wear cushioning/neutral shoes.

For an overpronator, the foot rolls inward more than is ideal because the foot and ankle can't adequately stabilize the leg. Because the ankle collapses inward, more of your weight is on the inside part of your foot, and you push off the ground using your big toe and second toe rather than distributing the force evenly across the ball of your foot. Overpronation is a major cause of running-related injuries. If you overpronate, you'll need a stability shoe, and if you overpronate a lot, you'll need a motion-control shoe.

For an underpronator, which is much less common, the foot doesn't roll inward enough after the outside of the heel lands. Consequently, the outside of your foot takes the brunt of the impact. Because your foot remains on its outside edge, you push off the ground using the smaller toes on the outside of your foot rather than distributing the force evenly across the ball of your foot. This can also cause injuries.

If you've never run before and have no idea how much your feet pronate when you run, go to a specialty running shoe store and have them watch you run to determine which shoes you should buy.

CUSHIONING/NEUTRAL SHOES

Cushioning shoes (sometimes called neutral shoes) allow your foot to pronate naturally to absorb shock upon landing. They're best suited for runners with normal to high arches because normal- to high-arched feet typically don't overpronate. They have minimal medial (arch-side) support, which you can see by the shoe's curved last—the mold around which a shoe is constructed. Cushioning shoes are distinguishable by the rubber on the medial side; it's compressible and is usually white. If you have a normal or high arch, pronate a normal amount, or even under-pronate, you should get cushioning/neutral shoes.

STABILITY SHOES

Stability shoes allow only limited pronation while retaining some cushioning characteristics. They're best suited for runners who have normal to low arches and mild to moderate over-pronation. You can tell a stability shoe by its added material on the medial side, which is firmer to the touch. If you have a normal or low arch and overpronate slightly, you should get stability shoes. Many overweight runners get stability shoes for the extra support; however, you may only need the extra stability if you overpronate.

MOTION-CONTROL SHOES

Motion-control shoes do exactly what their name implies—they control your foot's motion. They're best suited for runners with flat feet and severe overpronation. They have a straighter last than cushioning and stability shoes and contain a much firmer material on the medial side that's usually of a darker color than the rest of the rubber cushioning. If you have a very low arch (flat feet) and your foot rolls inward so much that it looks like it's about to fall sideways off a cliff, you should get motion-control shoes.

TRAIL SHOES

Trail shoes are specifically designed for running on trails. They have more support than road-running shoes and greater traction on the sole, and they're a darker color given how dirty they get when running on trails. Almost all trail shoes fall in the stability shoe category because of the extra stability needed on uneven

TIPS WHEN BUYING RUNNING SHOES

Don't think that more expensive shoes are better shoes. Buy shoes that are right for you regardless of price.

Match the size, width, and shape of the shoes to the shape of your feet. Don't try to fit a round peg into a square hole.

Make sure the shoes don't cause pressure points or squeeze your toes. Wiggle your toes in the shoes to make sure they can move around. Your shoes shouldn't compress your toes; they should allow for freedom of movement. Pressure can lead to blisters.

Buy shoes later in the day or after running, when your feet are slightly swollen.

Try on both shoes. There may be something in the right shoe that you don't feel in the left shoe. Both shoes need to feel comfortable.

When trying on shoes, wear the same type of socks that you wear when you run. The more you can re-create your running conditions in the store, the better the shoe fit will be.

Run in the shoes while still in the store. Shoes often

trails. However, you can still run on trails in cushioning/neutral shoes.

MINIMALIST SHOES

In response to the observation that many of the world's best runners grow up in poor countries running barefoot and the growing

feel very different when walking around the store versus actually running in them. You often feel things when you run in the shoes that you don't feel when you walk in them.

There should be a finger-width distance between your toes and the end of the shoe because your feet swell slightly when you run. Your toes should never touch the front of the shoes.

Buy shoes that breathe. Sweaty feet don't just make your shoes smell; they can also cause your feet to get hot, which is uncomfortable and can cause blisters.

Wear the shoes only to run. No matter how proud you are of your new shoes and your commitment to run, running shoes are best reserved only for their intended purpose.

Buy a couple pairs of shoes and alternate wearing them. Doing so lengthens the life of the shoes.

When you buy new shoes, keep the old ones to run in on rainy days.

Change your shoes after a few hundred miles because they lose their shock-absorbing abilities.

popularity of the (false) argument that shoes themselves cause injuries to runners because they force you to land on your heel, shoe companies have started developing "minimalist" shoes. As their name implies, these shoes have very little cushioning or support and a low or even zero heel-to-toe drop height to mimic barefoot running.

Some people argue that minimalist shoes decrease the risk of injury by altering the way your feet strike the ground and reducing your contact time with the ground. Cushioning shoes have a lot of padding in the heel, which promotes landing on your heel first. When you run barefoot or with minimalist shoes, you land more toward your forefoot than on your heel and spend less time on the ground. Proponents of barefoot running argue that it's a more "natural" way to run because that's the way our ancient ancestors ran. Although minimalist shoes and barefoot running do change how you run, whether they actually reduce injuries in runners is questionable. Currently, there is no research to support that minimalist shoes reduce the risk of running-related injuries.

Where your foot lands in relation to your hips matters more than which part of the foot touches the ground first.

Unless you're a very efficient runner to begin with, running in minimalist shoes or running barefoot is not a good idea. As an overweight runner, stick with running shoes that give you a lot of cushioning and support. Once you lose weight and get used to running, or as an intermediate or advanced runner, if you want to give minimalist shoes a try, I recommend using them to strengthen your feet by first walking around in them and then running in them only a few minutes a few times per week. Minimalist running shoes must be used very deliberately, progressing only a few minutes at a time.

APPENDIX B:
TECHNOLOGY TO
KEEP YOU RUNNING

WHEN IT COMES TO RUNNING, I've always been a purist. All I need is a pair of running shoes, the open road, and my own imagination. Perhaps that's because I grew up a runner before technology and moisture-wicking fabrics. Running used to be so simple—just open your front door and start running. Now, there's everything from GPS watches to iPods to keep you motivated to run.

Truth is, you don't need anything fancy to start running; but if you have the interest, there's almost no end to the technology that can enhance your running experience:

◆ **Running watch:** The most basic technology for runners, a running watch with a stopwatch lets you know how long you've been running and gives you exact times for your interval workouts. Get a watch with a rubber or Velcro band that stands up to sweat.

◆ **Heart rate monitor:** Checking your heart rate is a great way to determine whether you're running at the right intensity. Heart rate monitors come in a variety of styles. Some give you only your average heart rate for the whole run; some give you the high, the low, and the average; and others allow you to set a target heart rate range and beep when you go below or above that range. This latter option is great for beginners who need extra guidance on how fast to run.

◆ **GPS watch:** If a stopwatch and heart rate monitor aren't enough for you, a GPS watch has it all and then some—stopwatch, timer, heart rate monitor, instantaneous and average pace per mile, and distance covered. Some models come with a computer connection that allows you to upload the data from your workouts onto your computer, where you can generate graphs of all the numbers.

◆ **Apps:** There are a number of running apps to choose from to keep you motivated while you run, including RunKeeper, to track your runs and chart your progress; Couch-to-5K, which has preset 30-minute workouts to prepare you to run a 5K in 9 weeks; MyFitnessPal, to keep track of calories in your food log; and MapMyRun, which stores all of your running routes and maps out a course for you if you don't know where to run.

◆ **iPod or MP3 player:** If you can't stand the thought of running alone or while listening to your running partner drone on about his kids' grades in school, you can run with an iPod or MP3 player and listen to just about anything you want—music, a podcast, a favorite movie or radio program, or an audio book. Just don't get hit by a car while you're listening to Madonna through your headphones.

◆ **Moisture-wicking T-Shirt:** Throw away the 1980s cotton T-shirt and go for a moisture-wicking T-shirt instead, such as one made from Dri-FIT fabric, which wicks moisture away from your skin and keeps you cool. When it's really hot, wear a light-colored shirt that reflects the sun.

◆ **Sports bra:** Running presents a whole new challenge to well-endowed women. Get a bra that provides support, stability, and comfort. Choose fabrics like spandex, which provides stretch where needed, and breathable materials like Coolmax and Supplex, which wick away moisture and keep you dry. If you have small- to medium-sized breasts, get a compression sports bra, which holds your breasts close to your chest, restricting their movement when you run. If you have large breasts, select an encapsulation sports bra that limits the motion of your breasts by closely surrounding and separating each breast. Try on several sizes to find the one most suited to your body. Many specialty stores offer bra fittings for women with special needs. A bra with wide straps and a wide bottom band won't dig into your skin, provides the best support, and minimizes bounce as you run. A racerback- or T-back-style bra provides maximum freedom of movement. Avoid bras with inside seams that cause chafing.

ABOUT THE AUTHOR

A RUNNER SINCE AGE 11, Dr. Jason R. Karp is one of America's foremost running experts, an entrepreneur, and the creator of the Revo$_2$lution Running™ certification. He owns Run-Fit, LLC, the premier provider of innovative running and fitness services. He has been profiled in a number of publications and is the 2011 IDEA Personal Trainer of the Year (the fitness in-

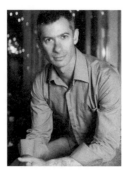

dustry's highest award) and 2014 recipient of the President's Council on Fitness, Sports & Nutrition Community Leadership Award.

Dr. Karp has given dozens of international lectures and has been a featured speaker at most of the world's top fitness conferences and coaching clinics, including Asia Fitness Convention, Indonesia Fitness & Health Expo, FILEX Fitness Convention (Australia), U.S. Track & Field and Cross Country Coaches Association Convention, American College of Sports Medicine Conference, IDEA World Fitness Convention, National Strength and Conditioning Association Conference, and CanFitPro, among others. He has been an instructor for USA Track & Field's highest-level coaching certification and for coaching camps at the U.S. Olympic Training Center.

A prolific writer, Dr. Karp has more than 200 articles published in numerous international coaching, running, and fitness magazines, including *Track Coach, Techniques for Track & Field and Cross Country, New Studies in Athletics, Runner's World, Running Times, Women's Running, Marathon & Beyond, IDEA Fitness Journal, Oxygen, SELF, Shape,* and *Active.com,* among others. He is also the author of seven other books: *The Inner Runner, 14-Minute Metabolic Workouts, Running a Marathon For Dummies, Running for Women, 101 Winning Racing Strategies for Runners, 101 Developmental Concepts & Workouts for Cross Country Runners,* and *How to Survive Your PhD,* and is the editor of the sixth edition of *Track & Field Omnibook.*

At age 24, Dr. Karp became one of the youngest college head coaches in the country, leading the Georgian Court University women's cross-country team to the regional championship and winning honors as NAIA Northeast Region Coach of the Year. He has also coached high school track and field and cross country. His personal training experience ranges from elite athletes to cardiac rehab patients. As a private coach, he has helped many runners meet their potential, ranging from a first-time race participant to an Olympic Trials qualifier. A competitive runner since sixth grade, Dr. Karp is a nationally certified running coach through USA Track & Field, has been sponsored by PowerBar and Brooks, and was a member of the silver medal-winning United States masters half-marathon team at the 2013 World Maccabiah Games in Israel.

Dr. Karp received his PhD in exercise physiology with a physiology minor from Indiana University in 2007, his master's degree in kinesiology from the University of Calgary in 1997, and his bachelor's degree in exercise and sport science with an English minor from Penn State University in 1995. His research has been published in the scientific journals *Medicine & Science in Sports & Exercise, International Journal of Sport Nutrition and Exercise Metabolism,* and *International Journal of Sports Physiology and Performance.*

INDEX

Note: <u>Underscored</u> page numbers indicate boxed text.

MARVEL

SPIDER-MAN

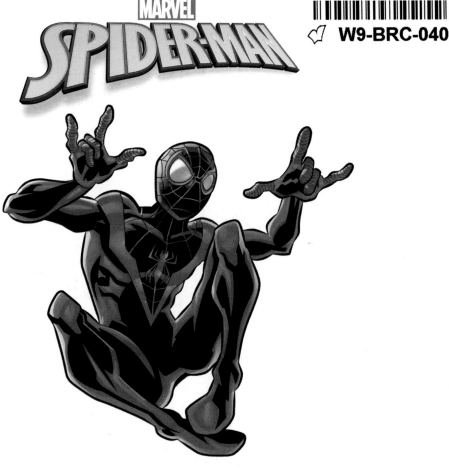

THIS IS MILES MORALES

Adapted by Alexandra West

Illustrated by Aurelio Mazzara and Gaetano Petrigno

Painted by Jay David Ramos

Based on the Marvel comic book character Miles Morales

MARVEL

Los Angeles
New York

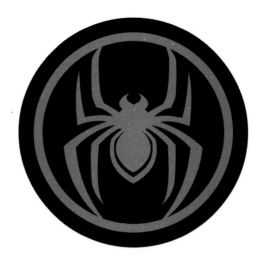

MarvelHQ.com

© 2018 MARVEL

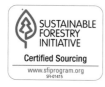

SUSTAINABLE
FORESTRY
INITIATIVE

Certified Sourcing

www.sfiprogram.org
SFI-01415

Printed in the United States of America
First Edition, October 2018 10 9 8 7 6
Library of Congress Control Number: 2018949011
FAC-029261-19347
ISBN 978-1-368-02863-9

This is Miles Morales.

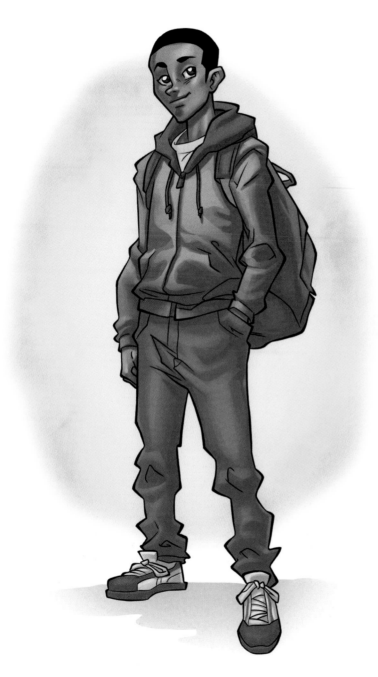

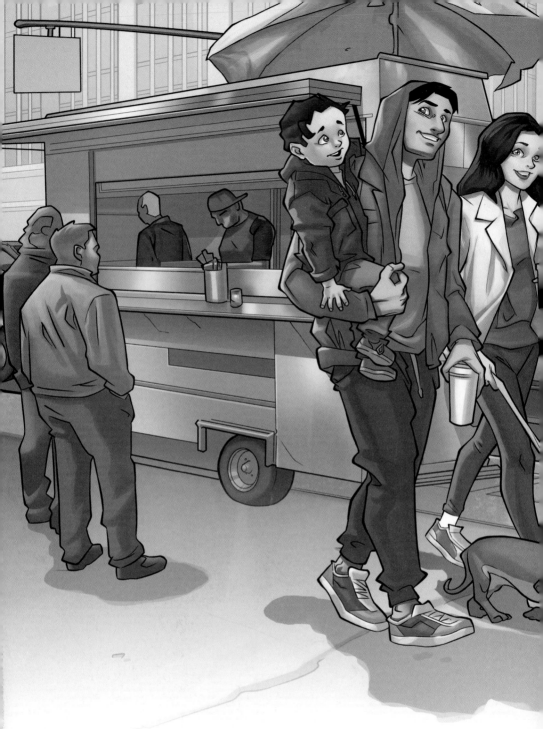

Miles Morales
lives in New York.

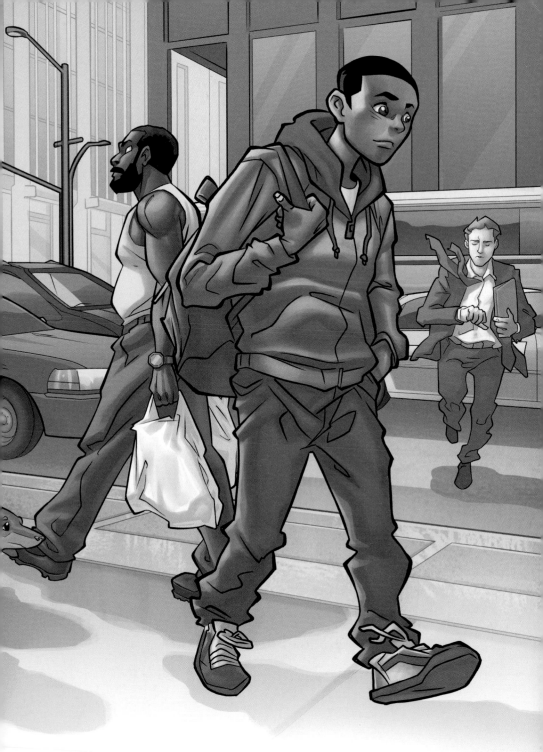

He is a
normal kid.

Miles Morales goes
to school.

He is very smart.

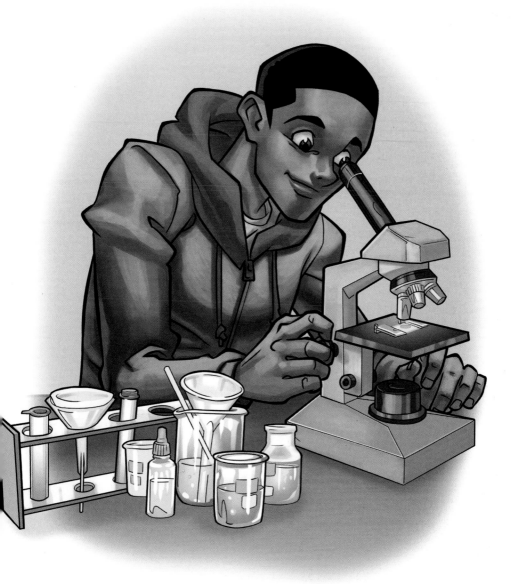

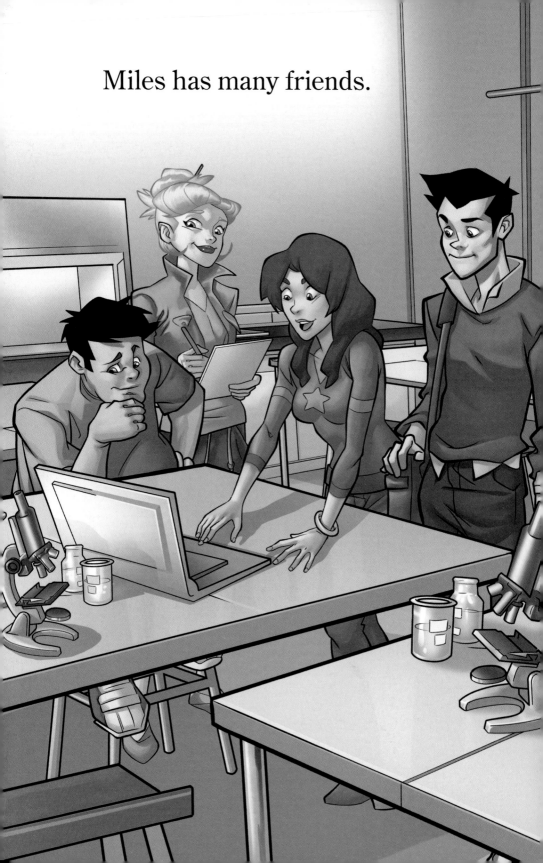

Miles has many friends.

He is friends
with Peter Parker.

Miles does not know that
Peter Parker is Spider-Man!

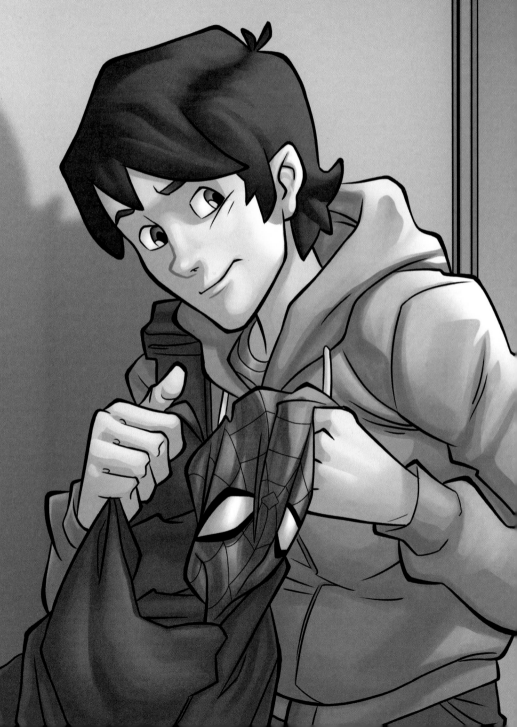

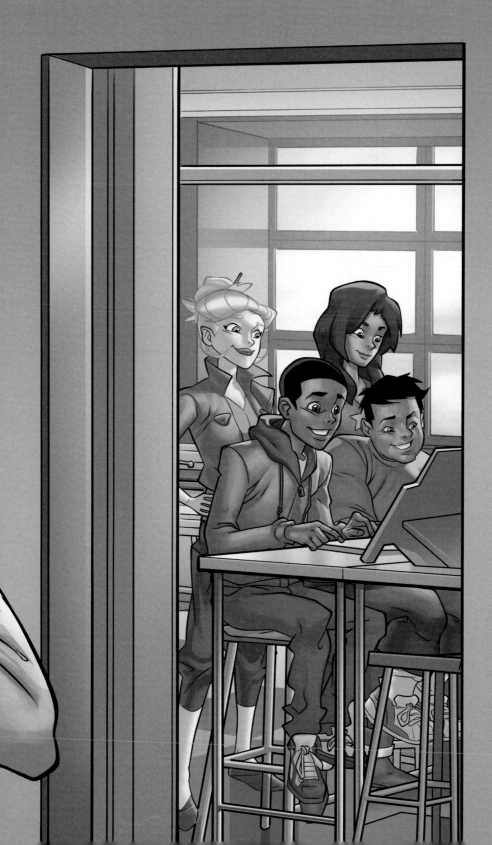

One day, Miles follows
Peter Parker.

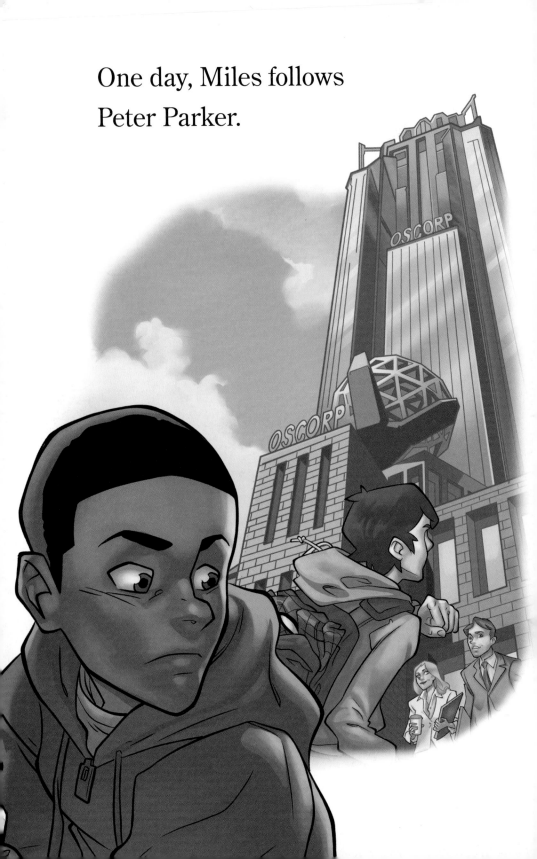

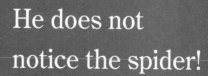

He does not
notice the spider!

The spider bites
Miles Morales!

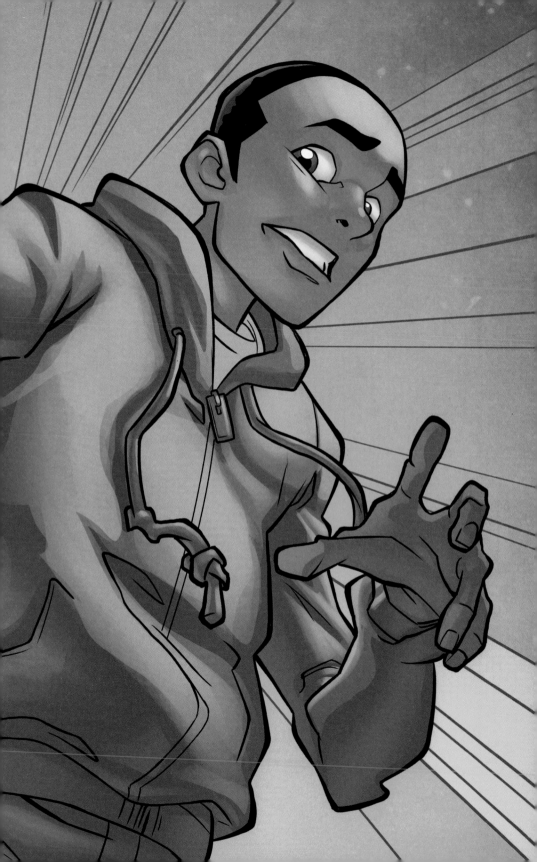

Miles gets super powers.

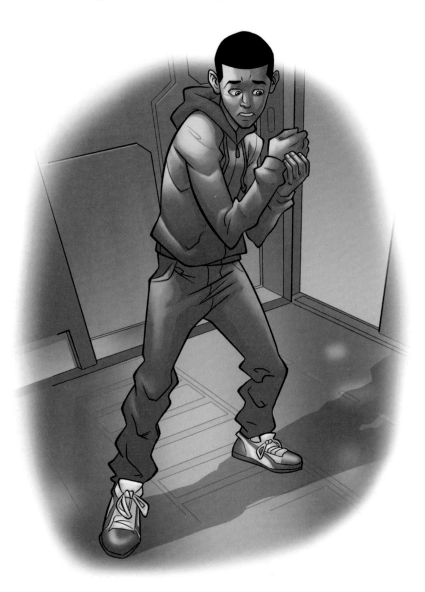

Miles gets spider powers!

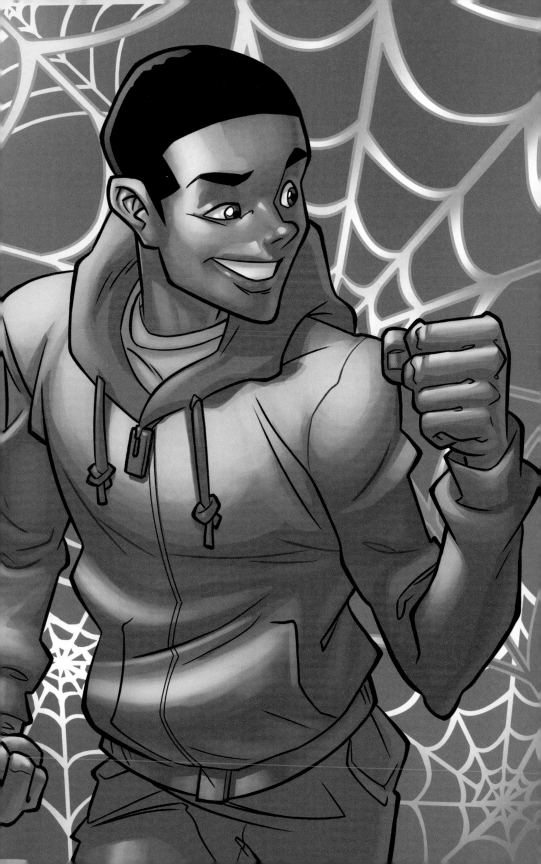

Miles can do
everything Peter can do.

He is strong.

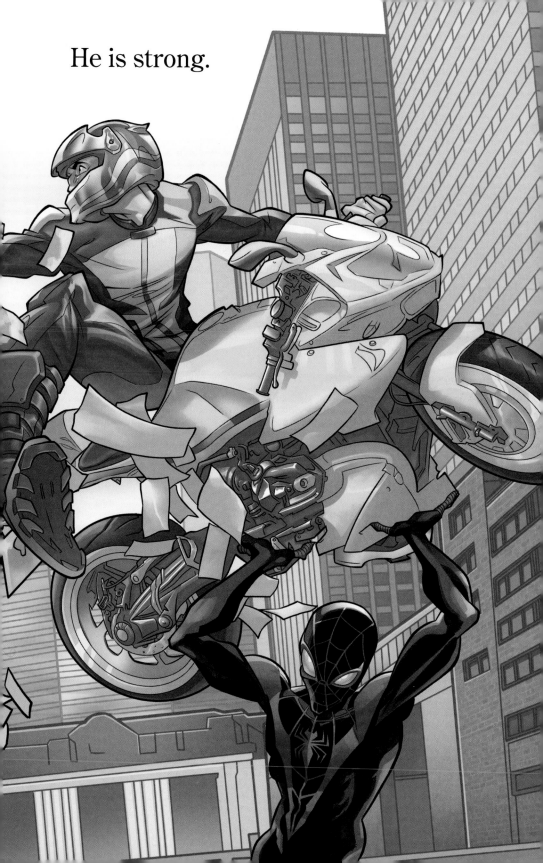

Miles can climb.

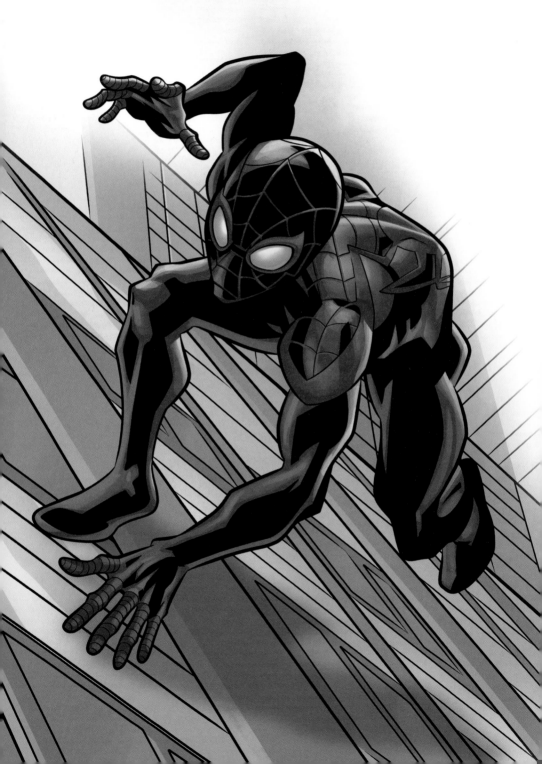

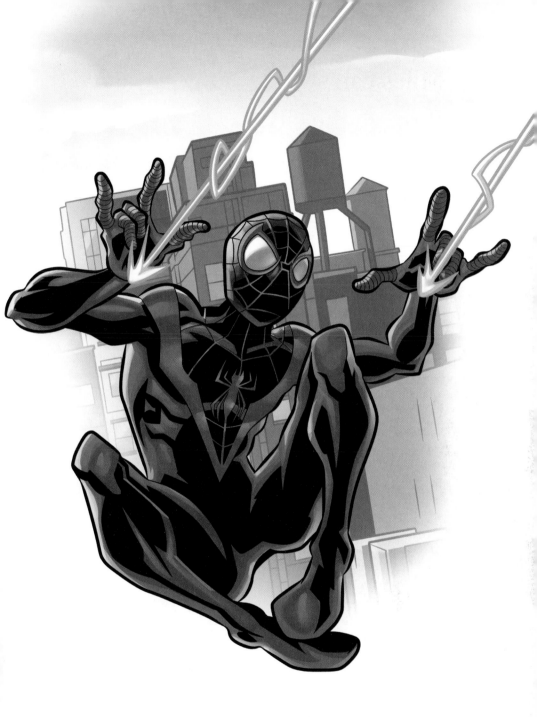

Miles can shoot webs.

Miles can swing
through the city.

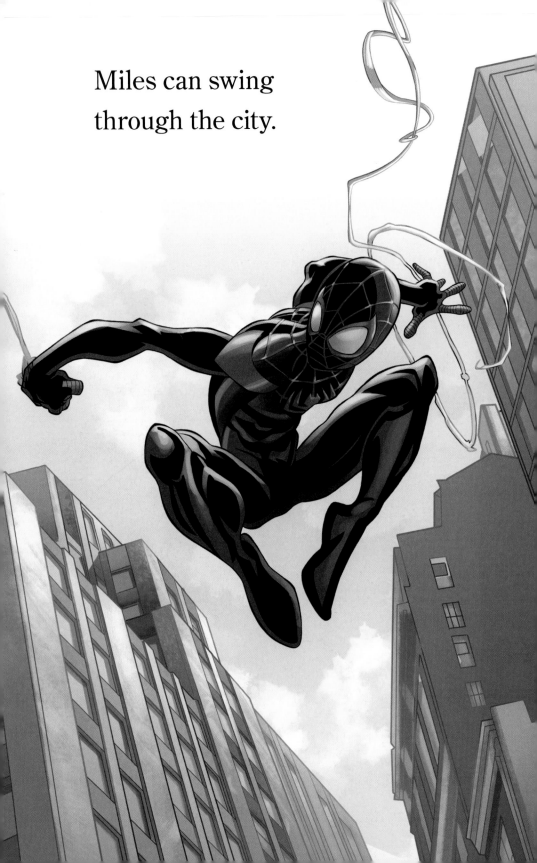

Miles has spidey senses.

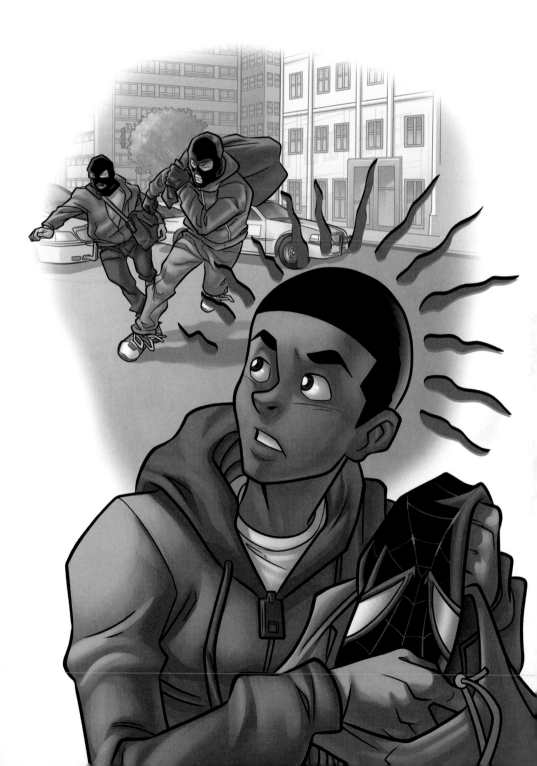

Miles can also do
things Peter cannot.

He has a venom strike.

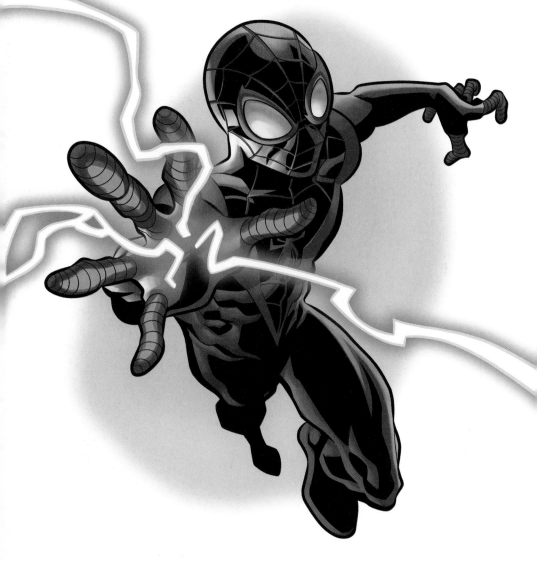

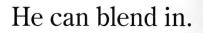

He can blend in.

Miles uses his
powers for good.

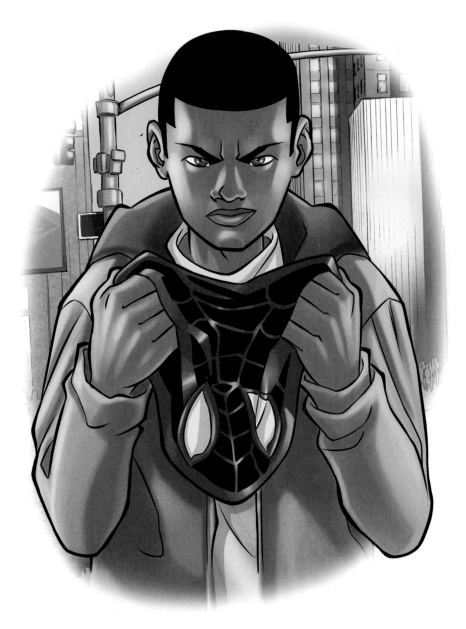

Miles and Peter
work together.

They fight villains!

Miles and Peter defeat villains!

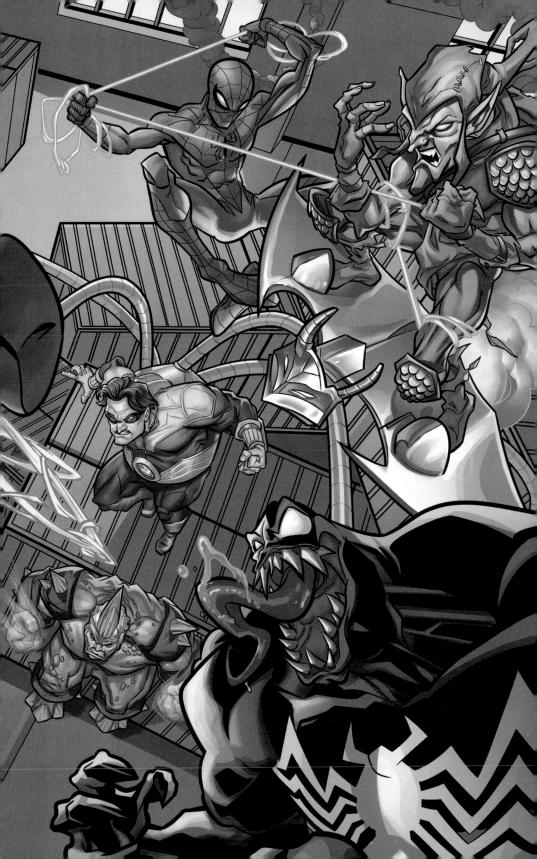

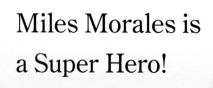

Miles Morales is
a Super Hero!

He helps Peter Parker
protect the city.

Miles Morales
is Spider-Man!

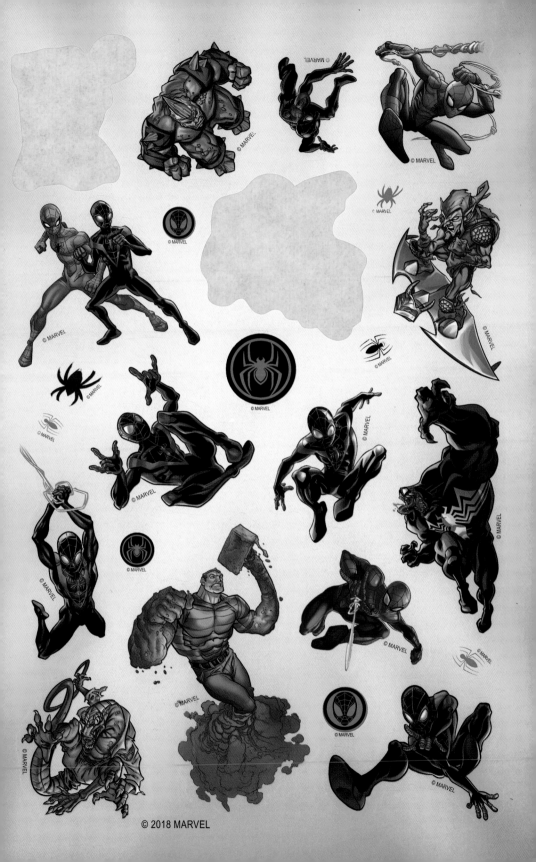